LABORATORY INSTRUMENTS OPERATION & MAINTENANCE

LABORATORY INSTRUMENTS OPERATION & MAINTENANCE

DR. SUSHANT PUNEKAR
M.Sc., Ph.D.
GOVERNMENT AUTONOMOUS P.G. COLLEGE,
CHHINDWARA (M.P.) 480002

BIOTECH

2012

BIOTECH BOOKS
NEW DELHI

ISBN 978-81-7622-245-7

Published by
BIOTECH BOOKS
4762-63/23, Ansari Road, Darya Ganj,
New Delhi-110002 (India)
Phone: 23262132
E-mail: biotechbooks@yahoo.co.in

Laser Typesetting by : Deep Graphics, Delhi

PRINTED IN INDIA

CONTENTS

PREFACE

The sophistication in instrumentation over the years has necessitated the knowledge in traditional areas like design of optical components, optical filters, photoelectric sensors, thin film deposition techniques, skills in handling high pressure cylinders and flames, discharge lamps, followed by electronic circuits, displays / readout systems, microprocessor/ micro-controller and use of modern test and measuring instruments. The successes in effective troubleshooting measures depend upon adequate use of knowledge and skills in these areas. With heavy emphasis in curricula and teaching for both undergraduates and post graduates for theoretical formulations in science subjects, the art of experimentation has suffered irreparably. Repairing, servicing and maintenance of instruments is a serious problem in educational sector all over the country and additionally the problem is compounded by short of grant- in –aids from state government and scientific establishments. There has been little understanding in educational sector as regards to instrument maintenance that deterioration, decay, obsolescence are inevitable and universal consequences of ageing process and aim of maintenance is to slow down these effects. We also do not recognise that failure to provide effective maintenance programme increases operating costs, reduce competitiveness and necessitates early investment in new systems

/ instruments. Operating on this basis alone, no educational institution can remain viable without looking at appropriate maintenance programme or strategy.

There is also another reason for the failure of effective strategy. One, there is apparent lack of appreciation of real needs for maintenance. Secondly, there is an apparent misconception that maintenance is secondary rather than a central factor in investment decisions. Also acquisition of new instruments is not accompanied by taking account of local conditions. This hampers maintenance and poor economy followed by weak engineering manufacturing base adds fuel to the problem. This weakens the ability of educational institutions to influence the range and type of instruments leading to the dependency syndrome of foreign firms. Establishing / commissioning of new instruments facilities even in these hard times of economy slow down is considered as an index of success without understanding that services with the time turns into frustration due to debilitating consequences of prolong neglect. One has also to recapitulate that in a globalized environment in which we live, the profit and losses are to a large extent, determined by the quality and effectiveness of maintenance. The dependability and high degree of availability are a function, of how well the maintenance operations are performed.

Hence the mission of maintenance is to provide optimum utilization of technician / scientist / teacher, materials, money and instruments. It is accomplished by, guaranteeing unlimited availability of facilities and instruments, preserving the capital investment, creating absolute reliability of facilities and instruments, ensuring the process operates within statistical control, replacing and rebuilding expanded capacity. Finally the, way to solve problem of maintenance passes through nature of faults, equipment failures, causes of failure, production deficiencies, trouble shooting, preventive maintenance and personal safety. This all chapters of the book will discuss these aspects.

The book is written in a lucid manner and the subject to instruments are divided into twenty chapters and the chapters are Opto- Analytical Instrument Maintenance, Optical Microscope, Maintenance of Optical Microscope, Maintenance of Optical Instrument, UV-Visible Spectrophotometer, Application of UV-Visible Spectrophotometer, Spectrofluorimeter, FTIR Instrumentation and Basic Concepts, Application of FTIR Spectroscopy, Flame Photometer, Nephalometer and Turbidimeter, Refractometer, Polarimeter, pH Measurement, Conductivity Measurement, Centrifuge, Balances, Single Pan Balance, Projectors, Microtome, Oven, Incubators, other Heating Instruments. All these instruments are mismanaged due to lack of skill towards scientific operation and proper handling of digital functions to evolve an approach towards a right maintenance of the sophisticated instruments. These are serious operation problems and most of the operators are not used even for calibration and error due to calibration. The aim of this book is to provide its readers an acquaintance of the proper operations and maintenance of sophisticated instruments.

In preparation of this resource package manual in this book form, I have become greatly indebted and needless to say that we took the help of large number of persons in this venture, therefore, it is not possible to acknowledge them individually and we owe our thanks to all of them to give final shape to the book. But, I wish to express my thanks to principal, a number of professors, colleagues and friends for their help and cooperation. I am grateful to Mr. Sunil Mittal publishers M/s Biotech Books, Delhi for taking special interest and efforts in the publication of this book without whose interest and endeavour this work would never have reached into the hands of the reader in such a present shape.

August, 2011

Sushant Punekar
Assistant Professor (Zoology)
Govt. Autonomous Postgraduate College,
Chhindwara (M.P.)

LIST OF CONTRIBUTORS

A.M. Narsale, Director, Western Regional Instrumentation Centre (WRIC), University of Mumbai, Mumbai

R.D. Tewari, Technical Officer, Western Regional Instrumentation Centre (WRIC), University of Mumbai, Mumbai

Sushant Punekar, Assistant Professor (Zoology), Govt. Autonomous Post Graduate College, Chhindwara (M.P.)

U.K.Jain, Professor (Physics) & Principal, Govt. Autonomous Post Graduate College, Chhindwara (M.P.)

Satish Shukla, Central Poultry Diagnostic Lab, Jabalpur (M.P.)

P.R.Chandelkar, Principal, Govt. Degree College, Junnardeo, District Chhindwara (M.P.)

S.R. Nawange, Fungal Disease Diagnostic & Research Centre, Jabalpur (M.P.)

LIST OF CONTRIBUTORS

ABBREVIATION

OAI	–	Opto-Analytical Instruments
GLP	–	Good Laboratory Particles
GALP	–	Good Automated Laboratory Practice
RP	–	Resolving Power
NA	–	Numerical Aperture
UV	–	Ultra Violet
NIR	–	Near Infrared
FIR	–	Far Infrared
RLD	–	Reciprocal Linear Dispersion
SBW	–	Spectral Band Width
IR	–	Infrared
AA	–	Amino Acids
PMT	–	Photomultiplier Tubes
DSU	–	Data Station Unit
SIT	–	Silicon Intensified Target
CID	–	Charge Injection Device
CCD	–	Charge Coupled Device

TCSPC – Time Correlated Single Photon Counting

TAC – Time-to-Amplitude Converter

RF – Radio Frequency

HG – Harmonic Generator

SHM – Simple Harmonic Motion

FTIR – Fourier Transform Infrared

FT – Fourier Transform

ATR – Attenuated Total Reflectance

JTU – Jackson Turbidity Unit

NTU – Nephelometric Turbidity Unit

FTU – Formazin Turbidity Unit

TU – Turbidity Unit

RPM – Revolution Per Minute

RCF – Relative Centrifuge Force

PC – Poly Carbonate/ Personal Computer

OHP – Over Head Projector

DMD – Digital Micro Device

1

OPTO-ANALYTICAL INSTRUMENT MAINTENANCE

Electromagnetic radiation almost pervades all walks of our life and its spectrum consists of large number of wavelengths. The proper choice of wavelength region has led to the development of large number of opto-analytical instruments (OAI). Hence electromagnetic radiation is a powerful tool to extract the information about chemical, agricultural, environmental, ocean graphic samples. In the recent years, it has been possible to use electromagnetic radiation for metrology, process control and telecommunication instrumentation. Instrumentation making use of electromagnetic radiation has become complex additionally due to sweeping revolutionary developments in microelectronics. We now hare 4 bits device to 64 bit microprocessor / micro-controller and finally, different versions of PC to interface with OAI. It is now possible with fairly good accuracy to asses the impact of electromagnetic radiation on different type of samples by using powerful sensors, micro-controller / processors and PC. Almost all the parameters can be effectively controlled electronically. This has led to automation and user friendliness in OAI. The greatest advantage of use of electromagnetic radiation lies in its non-destructive character in the sense that sample is not destroyed in the process of investigation. The sample is further amenable to other investigation.

The sophistication in instrumentation over the years has necessitated the knowledge in traditional areas like

a. design of optical components
b. optical filters
c. photoelectric sensors
d. thin film deposition techniques,
e. skills in handling high pressure cylinders and flames,
f. discharge lamps, followed by
g. electronic circuits,
h. displays / readout systems
i. Microprocessor/ micro-controller and use of modern test and measuring instruments.

The successes in effective troubleshooting measures depend upon adequate use of knowledge and skills in these areas.

With heavy emphasis in curricula and teaching for both undergraduates and post graduates for theoretical formulations in science subjects, the art of experimentation has suffered irreparably. Repairing, servicing and maintenance of instruments is a serious problem in educational sector all over the country and additionally the problem is compounded by short of grant- in –aids from state government and scientific establishments. There has been little understanding in educational sector as regards to instrument maintenance that deterioration, decay, obsolescence are inevitable and universal consequences of ageing process and aim of maintenance is to slow down these effects.

We also do not recognise that failure to provide effective maintenance programme increases operating costs, reduce competitiveness and necessitates early investment in new systems

/ instruments. Operating on this basis alone, no educational institution can remain viable without looking at appropriate maintenance programme or strategy.

There is also another reason for the failure of effective strategy. One, there is apparent lack of appreciation of real needs for maintenance. Secondly, there is an apparent misconception that maintenance is secondary rather than a central factor in investment decisions. Also acquisition of new instruments is not accompanied by taking account of local conditions. This hampers maintenance and poor economy followed by weak engineering manufacturing base adds fuel to the problem. This weakens the ability of educational institutions to influence the range and type of instruments leading to the dependency syndrome of foreign firms. Establishing / commissioning of new instruments facilities even in these hard times of economy slow down is considered as an index of success without understanding that services with the time turns into frustration due to debilitating consequences of prolong neglect.

One has also to recapitulate that in a globalized environment in which we live, the profit and losses are to a large extent, determined by the quality and effectiveness of maintenance. The dependability and high degree of availability are a function, of how well the maintenance operations are performed.

Hence the mission of maintenance is to provide optimum utilization of technician / scientist / teacher, materials, money and instruments. It is accomplished by,

a. Guaranteeing unlimited availability of facilities and instruments.

b. preserving the capital investment

c. creating absolute reliability of facilities and instruments

d. ensuring the process operates within statistical control

e. replacing and rebuilding expanded capacity.

Finally the, way to solve problem of maintenance passes through

a. nature of faults

b. equipment failures

c. causes of failure

d. production deficiencies

e. trouble shooting

f. Preventive maintenance and personal safety.

This article will discuss these aspects.

1. NATURE OF FAULTS:

There are variety of faults that can occur into OAI. Most of the OAI have immunity from optical faults but should they recur then they are of serious types.

i. 10 – 20 % of the optical faults are due to chipping or breakage at an adge.

ii. 30 % of critical faults in optical components are due to scratch and stripe.

iii. 50 % of optical faults are caused to sudden change in pressure and temperature.

iv. 5 % faults exist due to defects in glass. This includes bubbles and striae.

v. Some faults are introduced in optical components due to action of chemical agents

vi. 20 – 25 % faults are also seen due to inhomogenity

vii. 90 % of the faults in optical part is due to dirt, dust which affects the image quality.

viii. A rare fault in optical component is also produced due to deposition of the water and moisture resulting into a stain.

ix. The most significant contribution to fault also occurs due to deterioration in coating on optical components. This results into loss of reflectivity or transitivity.

x. A curious fault in the optical component like achromatic lens happens due to air bubble being trapped between two layers.

xi. OAI with flame as facilitator for analysis of chemical samples also pose problems. These problems are mainly linked to burner assembly, chimney, improper use of compressor, improper handling of gas cylinders causing flash-backs. These problems are routinely observed in the instruments like atomic absorption spectrophotometer and flame photometer.

xii. Most of the faults in OAI also occurs due to failure of the sensors to respond to optical radiation.

xiii. Many times a failure or fault in OAI occurs due to discharge lamps / flash lamps or failure in electronic circuitry.

Additionaslly, each OAI is accompanied in the end by sophisticated electronic gadgetry. There are numerous possibilities for faults to recur. Only few faults which are routinely observed are given below,

xiv. 30 % faults in an electronic instruments occur due to blown up fuse, broken or shorted power cord, sticky panel meters and defective connectors.

xv. 20-30 % faults are also due to improper ground leads causing spurious artefacts in recording instruments.

xvi. 10-30 % electronic faults are also due to impoper environmental conditions.

xvii. 10-20 % electronic faults are repeatedly observed due to loose mechanical fixtures, knob handles, power sockets, PCB, loose contacts of IC/Valve.

xviii. 40% of electronic faults which are neither simple nor common e.g. burnt transformer and erratic performance.

xix. 90 % faults in electronic ciruits are due to improper knowledge of use of power supplies or uninterrupted power supply.

xx. 10 % faults which comes in the category of chronic are due to displays or failure of readout systems including UPS.

Inspite of all the faults listed above there are situations in which OAI as a whole shows its inability to function as per specification. These may be partial, complete, gradual or catastrophic failure often caused by open circuit or short circuit.

2. CAUSES OF FAILURE:

The failure to perform as per specification in OAI happens due to following reasons;

i. **Improper designs**: This refers unsuitable choice of components, insufficient performance testing.

ii. **Improper validation**: This is due to lack of inspection and good sampling test and refusal of instrument to behave as desired by designer.

iii. **Substandard tools**: The use of undesirable tools lead to the manufacture of sub-standard instrument. This often happens due to poor motivation, lack of skill and sense of involvement of scientific staff / technicians.

Much of the hassles and failure in OAI can be avoided if causes are known. This helps one to avoid unfavorable effects. No optical component can be free without scratch and pits. These are primarily linked to cleanings of hands, gloves and cleaning cloth and workman / optician. To a very large extent, unclean floor, ceiling fans, worktables contribute to the production of scratch and pit in an optical component. Scratches also occur Thus fault diagnostic essentially is the fault establishment, fault location and fault correction.

Hence, the troubleshooting in effect boils down to develop fault finding aids and to generate effective troubleshooting techniques. These are different for electronic parts and optical parts.

The troubleshooting techniques for optical components require an elaborate knowledge of optical glass, homogeneity, freedom from striae and bubble, optical constants and resistance to chemical action. One also requires familiarity with optical machines such as glass cutting / trepanning / grinding / polishing / centering edging machine, test plates, precision angle protector, spherometer and truing tools. Armed with familiarity of machines and knowledge of the glass one can restore any optical component to its original capacity. The restoration process involves following steps

a. cleaning of fractured optical component by xylene / benzene
b. sawing the component
c. trepanning
d. subjecting the fractured component to size (means required angles or dimensions)
e. fine grinding and smoothing while maintaining dimension
f. Polishing and finishing of components and finally centering and edging. These operations on optical machines enable one to restore the component to the large extent.

The optical components which require recoating is subjected vacuum evaporation only after proper grinding / polishing process. The component needs to be kept in the vacuum chamber using proper adapter. An evaporation process is carried out under the vacuum of order of 10^{-5} to 10^{-6} torr followed by silicon monoxide layer to ensure the stability.

The removal of fungus in optical component in general is accomplished by using solvents like benzene, xylene etc. without affecting the polish.

Only solution to remove stains is not to expose optical components to atmospheric corrosion.

The loss of homogeneity of order $\lambda/4$ over a given area always reduce visibility of optical system. The solution lies regrinding the polishing. It must be emphasized that to maintain irregularity of order of $\lambda/4$ in any given OAI is an uphill task and infact an art. Never touch any optical parts by hands and if dirt or dust is to be removed, it has to be done by soft camel brush.

Many OAI have multi-layer dielectric coated mirror to enhance their performance. The restoration of dielectric coating in most of the mirrors is a Herculean task due to thickness requirement of materials to be coated and number times a layer of $\lambda/4$ has to be deposited. Additionally, one has to ensure high vacuum and deposition has to be carried out only after ion etching. Generally, the restoration charges are high with least fidelity for future.

The task of restoration to original in case of optical components is more facilitated by proper choice of mounts. Once proper machining and dimensions are achieved, the failure in performance is easily mitigated. The faults due to pressure and temperature are easily addressed.

The protection from atmospheric / chemical attack to optical component in most of the cases is achieved by using silica gel and proper casing. This is the most effective way to stop malfunctioning of the optical components.

Most of the lamps used for generating specific spectrum are either filled with air or some kind of gas (HCL-Neon + materials, deuterium lamp – isotope of hydrogen gas). Each lamp has about 500 hrs. as a life time. These lamps have to be thrown out once this limit is crossed. The other measure being replacing inert gasses in lamps like HCL/ deuterium The process consists of evacuating the lamp to a pressure of 10^{-7} torr and introducing inert or required gas slowly via needle valve and igniting discharge to observe the operation. The stable discharge around 0.5 to 1 torr ensures proper operation and vacuum sealing is accomplished at this juncture.

Many times a blister in an achromatic lens occurs due to loss of balsam and misalignment. In such a situation, the lenses are subjected to gradual heating and separation and further coated with balsam. A proper alignment of the lenses gives restoration to the original. These defects are more encountered in a system like spectrophotometer or its improved versions.

Using flames as a process to dissociate chemical species is very common in OAI. Effective results for premix burners are possible only when it is not subjected to oxygen. A good design of burner always ensures that a small volume of gas is occupied by the mixed gasses and lessens the danger. The nebulisation of samples in atomiser-burner assembly is generally achieved by maintaining a minimum pressure of 10 psi and maximum of 30 psi. The remedial measure for failure in compressor lies in replacing air filters / inlet-outlet valves / diaphragms / ball bearing and buffer tank. A flicker less during cleaning of protective layer as shellac. Cleaning dust particles using handkerchief or piece of cotton also causes haziness.

The real cause of stain in optical components is due to atmosphere corrosion and also due to formation of polymer. Fungal growth on components also contributes to the haziness and loss of image quality. This is particularly true in case of optical microscopes.

The deterioration in optical coating occurs mainly in the instruments like spectrophotometer and chief cause is the interaction of chemical agents with film. It also depends upon the conditions during evaporation such as clean substrate, order of vacuum and thickness.

The success in getting good quality image to a large extent depends upon homogeneity over a given area of an optical component. Most of the components require homogeneity over a given area better than $\lambda/4$. The loss in homogeneity is mainly due to rubbing on optical surface by some other surface and also due to application of heat to optical components.

In OAI the image fidelity is lost immediately if proper care of mounting and assembling is not undertaken. This undermines the life time of the optical components.

OAI with flame as a means to identify chemical species is appropriate if one has knowledge about gas mixture and burning velocity. Each gas mixture is characterised by a specific range value of burning velocity. It is always within 1m / sec. At atmospheric pressure, a steady flame is possible if mixture moves at a speed 3 to 10 time the burning velocity. Higher gas velocities causes flame front to blow and lower one leads to flash back. This means gas pressure must be appropriate to burner channel. Again flash back can cause explosion and has to be avoided at all cost. The flashback occurs only when flame propagates within the burner. The failure can also result due to improper functioning of burner-atomiser assembly. A selective evaporation of solvent mixture (e.g. alcohol + water) in a premix burner may cause sample to remain in the unevaporated portion of drops. Similarly, clogging of solution in atomiser can lead to disfunctioning of atomiser assembly. All these can lead to flicker in the flame and shall not ensure rapid response to new samples.

Most of the OAI uses a monochromatic as wavelength sorter to select a particular analytical line blocking neighboring lines. This function to a large extent depends wavelength dispersing prism or light cut off element grating. The failure to deliver appropriate line can be attributed to improper choice of dispersing element or groove frequency of grating. This is also followed by dirt, chip in illuminated and telescopic optics. These failures can also lead to lowering of band pass.

A failure in photoelectric sensor in OAI is generally attributed to radiation fatigue, loss of electrical contact.

The failure of discharge lamps in OAI can be attributed on account of loss of vacuum, loss of electric contract and permeation of gases in atmosphere leading to non-ignition of lamps.

There has been little understanding at least in OAI that lack storage facility can be contagious to the working / operation e.g. a fungus develops within few hours on optical components particularly in coastal area due to careless storage facility. This may happen to microscope, spectrophotometer or for that matter to any OAI.

As far as failure due to electronics in OAI is linked mainly to improper choice of components, insufficient testing, non availability of sampling test, fault finding aids, improper artwork on PCB, poor motivation, lack of skill also adds to failure.

The reasons for a failure in a microprocessor kit may be following

a. IC's popping out of their sockets
b. making improper power supply connections also connecting higher voltage than the specified ones
c. over loading peripheral chips during interfacing with external devices
d. increase in temperature of the processor IC's or peripheral IC's caused due to high room temperature without sufficient cooling.
e. subjecting kit to heavy mechanical shock or vibrations.
f. operating kit in the vicinity of high electromagnetic signal area and lastly due to sabotage.

OAI in general uses either LCD or PC monitor as display of readings. The maximum failure that can occur in LCD display is the disorientation of liquid crystals due to heavy shock or vibrations.

4. REMEDIAL MEASURES:

The remedial measures mean that one has to isolate the faults and correct the malfunctioning of OAI such that it returns to its expected performance level i.e. repairing and restoring capacity that has deteriorated. Flame is possible by cleaning nebuliser due to salt deposits with the help of small wire. The capillary attached to atomiser as well as burner head in these OAI should be flushed with water daily. Most of pressure drops in compressor are attended by checking rubber o-ring of inlet-outlet valves. Some of these measures improves the task of decomposition of chemical species with flame as a facilitator.

Photoelectric or photo voltaic sensors used in OAI are very sensitive to the prolong exposure of optical radiation. This gives the fatigue to sensors and hence whenever not in use a shutter is provided in the instruments to avoid exposure of light. Once a sensor is out of order, very little can be done to restore to its original value. However, its capacity can be expanded in normal situations by appropriate cooling and providing μ - metal shield to avoid other effects.

OAI require a radically different approach for failure electronics. The fault tracing and diagnosis is almost impossible without proper servicing and maintenance manual containing diagram of the electronic circuits. Beside this, a standard test and measuring instruments is another important requirement. The common fault finding aids are,

a. millimeter (analog / digital)

b. oscilloscope

c. signal generator.

The trouble-shooting consists of adopting a functional approach. In such a approach the fault finding is accomplished in an order of merit viz. power supply, amplification, generation, transmission, conversions, logical manipulations and storage. The isolation of faults is also achieved by split half method using divergent paths, power supplies, convergent path and feedback path.

5. VALIDATION AND MAINTENANCE OF OAI:

So often after maintenance of OAI is carried out, a question is put forth how much deviation from standard measurements? This question can only be answered by understanding a process called validation. It is a process to verify that an OAI is doing what it has been designed to do reliably and accurately. The validation involves instrument validation and finally checking the entire system for compliance to system suitability parameters. It also involves Good Laboratory Particles (GLP). GLP means conditions under which laboratory studies are planned, performed, monitored, recorded and reported to ensure the quality integrity and validity of data obtained. It has also another dimension viz. Good Automated Laboratory Practice (GALP). This contains principles and guide lines to ensure integrity and traceability of computerised data. Lastly, a important link with maintenance of OAI is the traceability of data produced to international specifications. Hence, this issue is more linked to calibration. All these aspects should be taken into account before stating return to the standard measurements in OAI.

6. PREVENTIVE MAINTENANCE:

This is carried out to increase the system reliability by decreasing the chance of failure and providing better functional performance. It includes inspection, servicing, replacing defective parts, checking indications, checking meter / gauges / audio indicators also corrosion and dirt.

7. PROFESSIONAL QUALITIES AND WORK HABITS:

The failure of any OAI is a challenge to professional experience, technical knowledge and mental discipline. Sometimes maintenance of OAI becomes very frustrating to the extent it makes one mad. This is one area of instrumentation where success is most of the time elusive and also depends to large extent upon safe working habits. The area of operation for OAI must be clean and instrument must be switched off before replacing any optical / electrical / electronic component(s). Improper application of force on circuit boards or connectors can result into damage. All the parts which are removed must be collected in a container so that these are not lost. A care has to be exercised in an electronic equipment or part while opening. A accidental fall of screw not retrieved may result into short-circuit on operation. A special methodology or training is required to handle faults in microprocessor / micro-controller kit. Similarly PC maintenance requires a good knowledge of digital technology / VLSI and working of printers and keyboards.

It should be remembered that in any OAI, a great care has to be exercised of optical components. No optical component should be touched by hands or by sharp objects. Adequate precautions should also be taken for OAI with flame as a facilitator. Flash up should be avoided at all costs.

Lastly, for any kind of OAI, main danger is from hazard of electrical shock. Instrument operator / user must use a pair of dry sneakers with rubber sole and keep feet separated from ground. Always keep fingers away from the moving parts and mechanism.

2

OPTICAL MICROSCOPE

An unaided eye is capable of observing between the finer details up to 0.1 mm size object and cannot discriminate objects smaller than this. The microscope is essentially a device which magnifies the image to reveal finer details. The finest details to which a microscope can sort out is termed as its resolving power (R.P.). There is a general agreement on tube length equal to 160 mm. Similarly, standardization has been achieved in case of the distance from objective to the shoulder of objective set at 45 mm. Other standards include object to image distance set at 195 mm; objective shoulder to intermediate image at 150 mm.

INTRODUCTION:

No microscope to date has been found suitable for all types of work. The reason lies in the universal nature of the specimens examined with the microscopes. Biological microscopes are unsuitable for crystalline material. Similarly, polarizing microscopes do not possess high resolution.

In general, choice of the microscope depends on size, orientation, application and problem to be dealt with. We discuss the optical components in the light of particular needs.

STAND:

The stand supports the body tube; the view heads, the nose piece the stage and sub stage with all of its attachments.

BODY TUBES, HEADS, NOSE PIECES:

The body tube is a cylinder with a viewing head on the top and nose piece at the lower end. It may contain a Bertrand lens with an arrangement for centering by means of a knob, and facility to remove from optic axis. The body tube will also contain analyzer having provision for rotation and graduation and can be taken out from the light path. Polarizer, lenses and compensators are also introduced into body tube. These provisions make polarizing microscope very expensive compared to other microscopes.

Higher magnification can be achieved using zoom optics or lenses providing stepped up magnification. The rotating nose pieces are definitely superior to individual objective carries and faster and safer to use, as each objective is properly centered in the nose piece.

OBJECTIVES:

Objectives are the most important optical components of the compound microscope. They form the intermediate image of the object which is subsequently examined with ocular.

There are three versions of objectives. They are achromat, fluorite and apochromat. Most of the objectives contain achromat and are corrected for chromatic and spherical aberration for two wavelengths and one wavelength respectively. Achromats have good working distance and moderate numerical aperture (NA) and are relatively easy to manufacture. One requires special type of objective for polarized light work. These are absolutely strain-free and are carefully made by slow cooling of glass.

Fluorite objectives or semi-apochromatic objective are highly corrected the apochromatic. Chromatic and spherical aberration both are corrected for two wavelengths. As a result, one obtains higher NA resulting into higher resolving power, It is achieved by the use of fluorite which has a dispersion not obtainable in glass. Recently, synthetic fluorites have been used for making microscope objectives. They are excellent compromise between universal achromats and highly corrected apochromats.

Apochromats are highly sophisticated objectives corrected for two wavelengths for chromatic aberration and two wavelengths for spherical aberration. The NA is higher for same magnification and images are sharp.

In addition to these three types, objectives are also classified according to correction viz, plano to flat field objectives. These flatten the image correcting for the field curvature using additional lenses. They are very important in photomicrography.

In the choice of various objectives one can set a thumb rule ; higher the NA, lower the working distance available.

One of the important points to be noted regarding the oil immersion objective is the oil itself. It is not enough to match refractive index of fornt lens (usually 1.515). The dispersion of oil must be correct.

OCULARS:

In order to get good image, the oculars play an important role. They produce a virtual image of the objective's image when seen, visually or real when used photographically. Basically, ocular has two lenses, a field lens and an eye lens. The eys lens of highly corrected ocular has a doublet and or triplet. One of the salient features of oculars is to correct the aberration in the objective image.

It is absolutely essential to have one-to-one correspondence between ocular and objective and lack of it may introduce curvature.

Wide field oculars are mainly used for greater eye relief. Oculars for use in polarizing microscopes have a key so that they fit one way in the body tube. This arrangement ensures that the cross hairs correctly indicate the north-south/east-west, direction of the polars. In fact, it is a good idea to buy a graticule that combines cross hairs and an ocular micrometer on the same disc.

SUBSTAGE:

The sub stage consists of components below the stage viz, iris diaphragm, condenser and the mirror.

The condenser provides a cone of light which illuminates the specimen and is least understood of the components of microscope. If one is not aware of NA OF THE CONDENSER, PROBABLY ONE DOES NOT KNOW THE CORRECT ADJUSTMENT AND ITS USE. If one buys an ordinary condenser without specifying, one ends up with two lenses. Abbe type, and less likely three lens type. Mostly, all bright field condenser are two lens type and less likely three type.

Generally, two lens system of condenser forms an image of field diaphragm in the field of view somewhat fuzzy along with the coloured fringes. This is due to the chromatic aberration. Such condensers are of no use for colour photomicrography. Condensers that focus the light in one plane are required and are known as planate.

There may be three or four achromatic lenses corrected for chromatic aberration and in critical microscopy it may be six or seven lenses.

If one has choice for mount, one should buy centering mount. This type of mount allows one to align the condenser with the optic axis.

Strain-free condensers are particularly used for polarized light and long working distances and used for dark field, interference microscopy. Quartz condensers are particularly used for UV light.

A mirror is provided as a part of sub stage when in-built light source is not include. The usual diameter of the mirror is 50-52 mm with one side plane and other side concave. The plane side of the mirror is always used in conjunction with the condenser. The concave side for low NA objectives when a condenser is not used at all. Polarizing microscopes have a graduated rotating polarizer in the sub stage position.

STAGE:

Most of the stages are square although circular rotating stage is far more useful for orienting a specimen for visual examination and for photomicrography. Stage in polarizing microscopes not only rotate, but are also graduated in degrees, an essential feature for work with crystals. This type of stage rotates on ball bearing.

ACCESSORIES:

Among the most frequently used accessories to the basic microscope are attachable mechanical stage in the square or circular.

Reticules and graticules are used in conjunction with the ocular and at the diaphragm. These are engraved glass discs and are bought into focus with the use of eye lens. These are useful when measurements are to be taken.

Stage micrometers are nothing but ruled glass or metal plates, or reduced photographic scales of known length used for calibrating ocular micrometer.

Light filter are essential for visual microscopy as well as photomicrography. They are helpful for (a) adjusting colour balance (b) reducing intensity (c) increasing contrast (d) providing monochromatic light. They are particularly useful for determining refractive index and in phase contrast work.

LIGHT SOURCES:

One generally uses low voltage light sources. They are (a) tungsten filament lamp (b) quartz halogen lamp. Some microscopes have in-built light sources; for others a provision must be made for condenser system. For separate ligh sources, one must have adjustable diaphragm which does not change position when condenser is focused.

Quartz halogen lamps have been generally introduced by all manufacturers. They have sufficient light output and with a well known characteristic. Their disadvantage: lager amount of heat dissipation. This can be controlled by suitable design of lamp housings.

Other light sources are mercury lamp, 100 W, 12 v projection lamp, and xenon lamp. These are generally on higher side of cost economics.

PHOTO MICROGRAPHY:

Assuming one has a 35 mm camera, the simplest way to take a photo micrograph is to buy or make connecting tube for attaching the camera body without a lens to the body tube. Video microscopes are very popular and useful today for biological, Medical, Metallurgical, tool room and industrial laboratories.

CARE AND HANDLING OF MICROSCOPES:

Modern microscopes are robust, precision-built and require expert attention. With a little care, they normally give years of trouble-free service.

The optical system of the microscope is the most important part of the system, so the lenses and the slides should be kept clean at all time.

Dust and grease not only reduce transmission and clarity, but can add confusing artifacts to an image. Dust contamination can be minimized by keeping the microscope under a polythene cover when not used. Before use, the eyepiece and objective should not be touched with fingers. But if this happens, the lens should be cleaned with a soft tissue paper or cloth. If the lens is contaminated with grease, it should be cleaned with xylene.

If a lens or prism becomes damaged or dirt finds its way inside, it should only be serviced by a trained technical. To minimize dust entering the body tube and contaminating the backs of lenses, removal and interchanging of eyepiece and objective should be done if necessary.

Microscopes are fitted with multiple nosepieces so that three or more objectives can be kept on the microscopes at all times. If

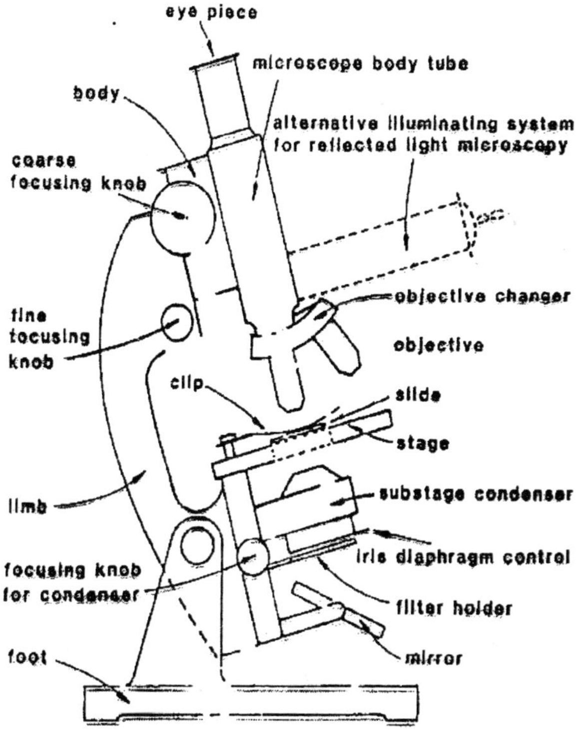

The Mechanical Construction of the Optical Microscope

a lens is used occasionally, it is better to remove it after use, clean and keep it in its storage or in a container. After use, clean the objective front lens, the condenser top lens and the slide carefully and thoroughly with a piece of cloth moistened with acetone or xylene. Focusing system should only be dismantled and lubricated top lens trained technicians. Stands and limbs are generally robust castings with enamel or hard synthetic coatings. If cleaning a necessary, wipe other with a damp cloth using a mild detergent.

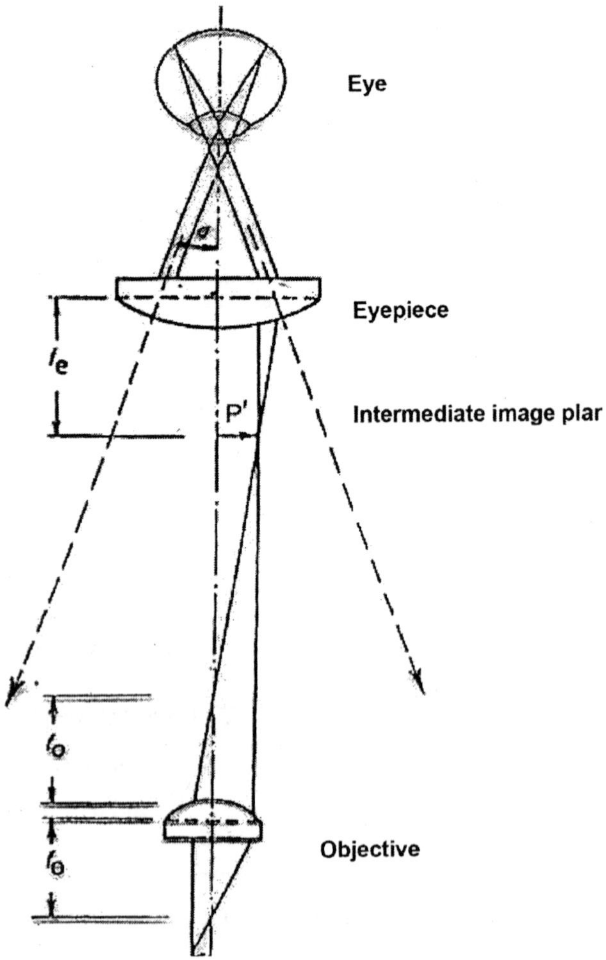

Microscope is an instrument, which enables us to see very small objects, which cannot be seen with an unaided eye. Generally our eyes are capable to see up to 0.1 mm, beyond this it is very difficult to see and that is why microscopes are very useful. Microscope is used to magnify the image of a small object with the help of a small objective lens kept towards the object and an eyepiece kept towards the eye in the microscope tube.

When our eye is unaided, the magnification depends upon the angle subtended at our eye is known as *viewing angle* and the size of the image is apparent. Two objects of different sizes viewing within the same angle have equal apparent sizes. The apparent size of an object can be increased, if it is brought closer to eye. But there is a certain limit to bring the object more close to our eye is known as the minimum distance of distinct vision and is approximately equal to 250mm. To increase the apparent size a lens can be used is known as magnifier or a simple microscope.

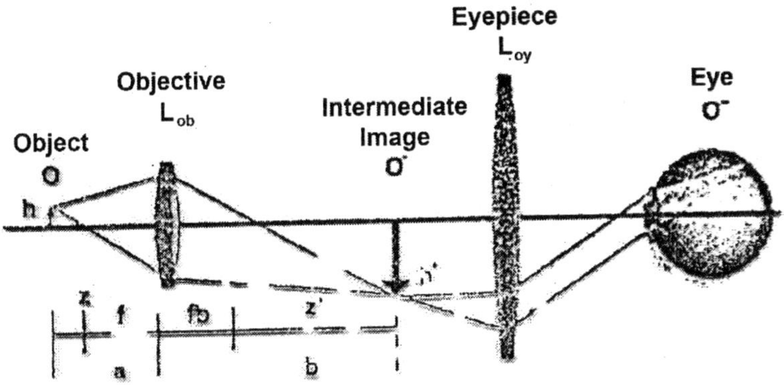

Magnification of objective:

$$M_o = (\frac{V_o - f_o}{f_o})$$

Where, $v_0 - f_0 = t$ = Optical tube length.

Hence the magnification of objective is fixed and depends upon the focal length of the objective. Similarly, magnification M_e produced by the eyepiece,

$$Me = \frac{D}{fe}$$

Hence the total magnification produced by Microscope

$$= Mo \times Me = \frac{T \times D}{fo \times fe}$$

However.a tube lens is incorporated in microscope of Mt magnification, then the total magnification is = Mo × Me × Mt

Approximate values of Mo, Me and Mt are marked on the eyepiece, objectives and the tube lens mounts. If accurate value of magnification is required it must be measured by means of stage or micrometer eyepiece.

Limit of Resolution and Resolving Power:

The limit of resolution is the measure of ability of the objective to separate in the image individual, adjacent details that are present in the object; it is the distance between two points in the objects that are just resolved. The resolving power is the reciprocal of the limit of resolution and is expressed in the unit of line resolved per millimeter. Suppose a grating of ruling d is illuminated with an angle of incidence i, then,

Resolution of optical microscope is 200nM, 1nm= 10^{-7} Cm

$$\lambda = d\ sinsi_1 + d\ sin\ i_2$$

$$d_{min} = \lambda / 2sinsi_2 \text{ if } iI=i_2$$

Moreover the object space is filled with a medium refractive index n, the ave length of light in the medium is λ/n, therefore,

$$d_{min} = \lambda / 2\ n\ sinsi_2 \text{ (Diffraction Theory)}$$

$d_{min} = \lambda / 2\ n \sin a$ Where, 'n sin a' is known as Numerical aperture is one of the important characteristics.

$$d_{min} = \lambda / 2\ NA$$

Lord Rayleigh arrived at the criterion for resolution using a complimentary approach. Owing to diffraction, the image of a point of light is a point surrounded by concentric dark and bright rings, the intensities of which decreases rapidly. When the images of two points are brought sufficiently close together for their diffraction patterns overlap, the points cease to be distinguishable. Rayleigh assumed that this occurs when the separation of the points in the image is equal to the radius of the first dark ring of point 1 coincide with the central bright disc of point 2, and vice versa. Quantitatively this leads to an expression for the limit of resolution.

$$d_{min} = K\lambda / 2\ NA$$

where, 'K' has a value of 1.22 when the objective is filled with light from a suitable condenser. This value is close to that deduced from diffraction theory. From this equation it is easy to see that resolution can be increased either by increasing NA or by decreasing λ. Consequently, microscopes are usually equipped with objectives of NAs .1 to 1.30

Numerical Aperture: $N.A = n \sin\alpha$

Where, α is the angular aperture which is semi vertical angle of the cone of light entering into lens system.

Coherent and non-coherent light:

Geometrical optics enables us to understand the way in which a microscope produces a magnified image, but it tells nothing about the quality of the image that is formed. To understand this we must consider image formation in terms of wave theory of light. Separate waves of same frequency interfere, depending upon their phases, but waves with different frequencies and behave as if they were isolation. Rays which are able to interfere are known and coherent and those who do not known as non-coherent. The eye is able to distinguish differences in amplitudes because of intensity of a ray of light is proportional to the square of its amplitude. Eye can also distinguish wavelength due to its different colour but it can not distinguish differences in phase. Therefore, we wish to make use of the differences in phase to distinguish between different constituents in a microstructure, the difference in phase must be translated in the difference in amplitude. Truly coherent light, in which all the waves are exactly in same phase, is only obtained from individual atoms and from lasers. Fortunately the, the phases of rays emitted by an incandescent light source can be considered to combine to produce a composite waveform that is unique to the source of any instant, but waveform will vary with time. Hence, provided the source that the source subtends a small angle at the point of interest so that it approximate the point source, each ray from it will have an identical wave form and the beam can be regarded as being coherent: such sources are called compact sources. A compact source of monochromatic light radiation all directions light waves, which are all of the same frequency and which, are all in same phase. Thus at all points of a spherical surface having the source as its center, the waves will be in phase. Almost all-light sources in microscopy are of this kind, including widely used tungsten filament lamps, arc lamps, mercury lamps and xenon lamps. Even the traditional light source sun of this kind because it is so far away that it subtends only a very small angle at the point of interest. We consider any point on an object source emitting waves in all directions and there are so many such sources on an object. If all the waves leaving a point on the object could recombine a perfect image of the object could be formed. In practice it does not happen because many of the waves travel in different directions difficult to collect. Thus perfection of image depends upon the amount of light collected by the optical system; the rays are in focussed accurately and are in phase.

Thus phase relationship of the rays is especially important when they are coherent. When two coherent rays combine, the amplitudes of their waves are additive. Hence, since the brightness of the light is proportional to the square of the amplitude of the waves, when two waves are of equal amplitude are exactly in phase the brightness of the resultant wave is four times that of either of original waves. Conversely, when they are exactly out of phase, light is extinguished. On the other hand non-coherent waves do not interfere or combine. Thus when two non-coherent waves of equal amplitude propagate, the intensity is simply twice that of either of the original waves. When, in an image formed by coherent light, fail to remain in phase, the quality of the image deteriorates and diffract more than shorter ones. Since microscope images are formed by diffracted waves, it follows that the small points are more easily resolved by the light of shorter wavelength, (blue light), than by the longer wavelength (red). Consider a wide slit illuminated with coherent (monochromatic) light. As the light emerges from slit it spreads sidewise. When the edges of slit are brought closer the spread becomes greater and eventually light and dark bands appear on the either side of t the image or direct beam. In a similar manner when a pin-hole is illuminated the direct beam is surrounded by dark and bright concentric rings known as Airy disc. The direct beam is called zero order and the successive rings of the diffractive beams are described as 1st order, 2nd order and so on. This effect in a single slit can be transferred to two or more number of slits. Abbe's theory of microscope: Considering the case of image formation in a transmitted –light microscope. A transparent object A is illuminated by a collimated beam of light. Thus from point Po the objective lens will collect direct and diffracted light and they are also collimated and after passing through the lens the rays will come in focus in the back focal plane of the objective each beam forming the image of the light source. These images of the light source are Huygenian subsidiary sources, each of which sends out waves that form by destructive interference the image of point P_0 in the image plane I at point P_i. The subsidiary sources lie on the arc of a circle centered at Pi, so that all the subsidiary waves reach Pi in phase and reinforce each other. Thus there is produced a bright image of P_0 which is surrounded by dark and bright rings formed by the interference. The central bright dick is the true image of the object but the surrounding rings (bright) reduces the sharpness of the image.

Three main conclusions are drawn from the detailed theory. Firstly, at least two beams must be collected by the objective if the details of the image to be resolved, because at least two beams need for interference occur, if only direct beam is collected no detail can be seen in the image. Secondly, to form the best possible image the entire beam diffracted by the object ought to be collected by the objective and used to form the image.

PHASE CONTRAST MICROSCOPY:

Some specimens are unable to produce sufficient to enable the detail present in them to be visible in bright field illumination.

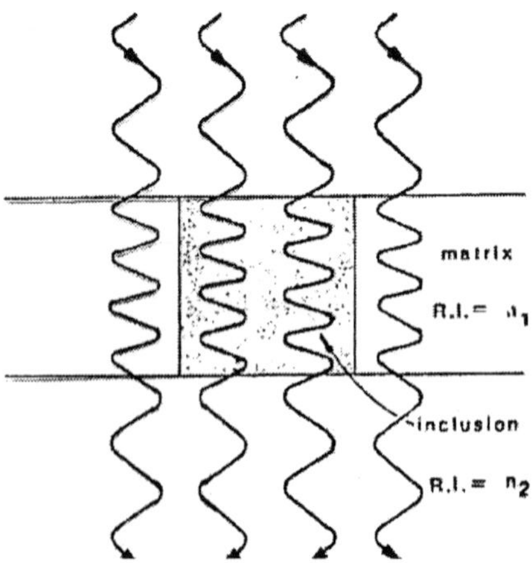

There are two kinds of specimen with which phase contrast microscopy may be useful. Firstly, transparent specimens that have regions of different optical density. Secondly opaque reflecting specimens that show small variation in surface level.

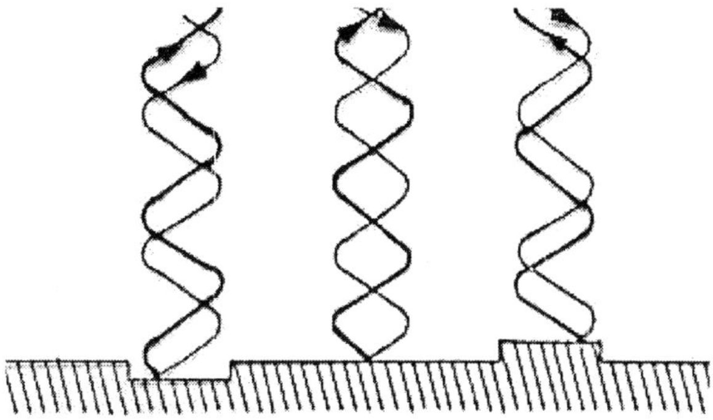

For first case as the as the beam passes through the specimen, the phase of rays passing through the inclusion lags behind that the rays passing through the matrix. When the two sets of rays which are of equal intensity, emerge from the specimen are out of phase by exactly half a wavelength and they interfere destructively causing the inclusion to appear dark, i.e. contrast is produced. However, in the specimen of normal thickness, the phase shift produced is usually an eighth. A quarter of an wavelength and a phase plate, that either accelerates or retards the phase of direct beam by a quarter of a wave length is used to increase the degree of interference between the beams and thus increase contrast. Same thing will happen for reflecting specimen if the surface is uneven.

The principles of reflected and transmission type phase contrast microscopes are same. In the latter case the annular diaphragm is located in the front focal plane of the condenser so that it will illuminate the specimen with a hollow cone of light. The condenser is focused so that the image of the annulus is formed at the back focal plane of the objective. A transparent phase plate carrying an annulus of same size as the image of the condenser annulus is inserted in this plane and it made to coincide exactly with it. The annulus of the phase plate retards or retards the phase of the direct beam, all of which is passes through it. Diffracted, refracted, and reflected pass the hole of the phase plate and most of them undergo no phase change because they don't pass through the annulus. Thus the direct and diffracted beam interferes to form the image.

For maximum contrast two beams must be of equal intensity and therefore the annulus of the phase plate is coated with some absorb and materials, like Antimony which reduces the intensity of the direct beam about 80% to match with the diffracted beam. The phase changing annulus may be either a grove in the glass, that reduces the optical path length through the glass thus, advances the direct beam, related to the diffracted beam, giving positive phase contrast or a transparent layer of dielectric material often magnesium fluoride, to retard the direct beam giving negative phase contrast. With transparent specimens, positive phase contrast causes areas of greater optical density that is greater R.I. or thickness, to appear darker than their surroundings and vice versa for negative phase contrast. Variation in optical thickness of about 3nm can be detected using positive phase plate in green light. The difference in optical thickness, t_0, is given by the equation,

$$t_0 = (n_1 - n_2)\, t$$

Where, n_1 and n_2 are the refractive indices of the constituents and t are the physical thickness of the specimen. Thus is a constituent in a slice of material 30μm thick is to be made visible by phase contrast, the difference between the R.I.s of the constituents needs to be only 10^{-4}. Thus the technique is useful for revealing subtle differences in R.I.s between constituents or regions within a specimen, as in organic polymers and glasses.

Unfortunately the images are formed are imperfect. The most pronounced blemish is the formation of bright haloes around constituents, owing to the direct and diffracted beams being imperfectly separated. In reflected light, phase contrast microscopy enables differences of surface level of 5-50nm to be distinguished, maximum contrast being obtained in the range 20-30 nm. However, adsorption and the halo effect may confuse the image. True phase contrast effects are identified by examining the feature, in turn, under positive and negative phase contrast conditions. If the feature changes from light to dark, or vice versa, on changing from one to the other, the effect is due to the phase contrast depressions appear darker than high spots and vice versa for negative phase contrast conditions. If the surface levels of features differ by larger amounts, e.g. about 100nm, the contrast may be reversed, but differences of this magnitude can be even seen in bright field illumination. In many cases the effects observed using phase contrast illumination depends more on absorption of light by the phase ring than its ability to shift the phase of the light. Thus the image may be regarded as being formed by the combination of phase contrast and opaque stop illumination.

INTERFERENCE MICROSCOPY:

Interference microscopy is based upon the principle of interference of light waves, which are out of phase by half a wavelength and interfere destructively. Phase contrast microscopy is a special case of it. The techniques of interference microscopy enable the variation of surface level observing the interference fringe pattern or contour.

Two-beam interferometry / Linnik interference microscope:

The simplest arrangement for two beam interferometer is an interferometer, in which a monochromatic beam of light is divided into two equal intensity perpendiculars to each other. One beam passes through the high power objective O and is focused on the on the specimen, while the passes through the matched objective O' and is focused on a metalized optical flat. The beam reflects and again interferes destructively in the front focal plane of the eyepiece if their phase difference is $n\lambda/2$. Where, n is an odd number.

MULTIPLE BEAM INTERFEROMETY:

A partially silvered reference plate is closely placed parallel to specimen plate and a well collimated monochromatic beam at normal incidence illuminates the specimen.

3

MAINTENANCE OF OPTICAL INSTRUMENTS

The process of maintenance of optical instruments/microscopes consists of four phases:

1. Pre-disassembly procedure
2. Disassembly, Overhauling, Repair and Re-assembly
3. Collimation
4. Removal of Parallex and Inspection

PRE-DISASSEMBLY PROCEDURE:

Before carrying out the repair work of an optical instrument, clean the work area, hands and keep every thing ready, like hand tools, cleaning materials, magnifiers, light sources etc. Cover the working area or table with a sheet of clean dry paper. Clean out side of the instrument with a clean cloth. One can use acetone or any approved dry-cleaning solvent.

Checking of optical system:

Because optical system constitutes the heart of an optical instrument, inspection of it is very important. The best method to follow in inspecting the optical system of an optical instrument is to point it towards an illuminated area and look. If the image is hazy or clouded, there may be some spots or dirt may be on the objective lens or on the prism of an optical instrument. It may cause a hazy or clouded image.

One can examine the color filters, objectives and eyepieces by rotating and holding one eye at a slight distance from the eyepiece. If there is not dirt, dust grease or oil and still the image is not sufficiently good, then one should check the mounts of the optical elements. If the mounts are loose, centering of the optical system may go off and that is why the image is not perfect.

If the field of view is not perfectly round, there may be a loose diaphragm inside the instrument. Check the antireflection coating on the coated optics by holding the component in daylight. If the coating is off proper thickness, the color of the reflected light is reddish-purple. If the coating is thin and not proper, it looks pale yellow and reddish brown. Fungus or deteriorated balsam can also create hazy image.

Reflecting surface of the prism, which is used for TIR is not coated as it may cause too much loss of light. Inspect prisms and mirrors for the sign of peeling and darkening of aluminum / silver coating.

DISASSEMBLY: (CARE & CAUTION)

a. When one disassembles an optical instrument, should not mix the parts of one instrument with other.
b. Keep the parts of one instrument in a separate box for proper identification.
c. Before disassembling one instrument, determine, whether push-fitted or threaded. One can use marking pencil for marking on the parts at the time of disassembling. This helps to identify the various parts.

Repair Tools for Disassembly /Assembly:

a. Grip-wrenches

b. Retainer ring wrenches

c. Set of screw drivers

d. Set of spanners

e. Allenkeys

f. Pliers

g. Files

Removal of Parts:

One can remove the parts using hand tools.

a. To avoid damages of optical parts remove them first.

b. Use proper tools; do not crush parts with wrenches.

c. If you could not remove a lens, cover it with a pad of soft cotton. Use wooden block to hold.

d. If a screw it tightened into a hole, loosen it with penetrating oil like kerosene or carbon tetrachloride.

Save the heads of the screws (Use extreme care and patience while doing this).

Clean all the parts check them and write the faults in detail in a notebook. Once you have cleaned and inspected the parts of the instrument, undergoing repair, follow either the procedures given below.

1. Repair and refitting the old parts.
2. Using a new part or replacement.
3. Manufacturing and refitting of new part.

Miscellaneous Repairs:

There may be a lack of lubrication or dirty lubrication, excessive or insufficient clearance, incorrect alignment in some optical instruments. One should follow the procedures given below:

a. Clean all the parts of bearing assembly and rack and pinion.

b. Try to assemble the various parts but do not force.

c. If there is excessive clearance in rack-pinion or bearings, put a very thin metallic foil under rack.

d. If there is insufficient clearance in rack-pinion or bearings remove or scrape away the high spot or file very carefully. Do not remove too much material.

Lens cleaning & Cleaning Equipment:

Syringe, camel hairbrushes, alcohol, medically pure acetone, lens tissue, absorbent cotton, wood / peg-wood stick. 'Teepol' is a grease-free detergent, can be used for cleaning. One can also use xylene.

Cleaning Glass / Optics:

a. Blow all coarse particles and remove the dirt with a syringe from the surface of the component.

b. Brush the surface with a soft brush using quick and light strokes.

c. If the size of the lens is large, one can use lens tissues damped with a few drops of acetone to remove the dirt and grease. Change the cleaning pads or swabs frequently. Use cotton, silk and lens tissues for small lenses.

d. Finish the cleaning of optics by using a pad with a few drops of acetone or alcohol.

Caution:

a. If you use a swab or pad moistened with acetone more than 20 sec. On an optical surface, it leaves a film or water mark on the surface. Avoid this any cost.

b. Acetone is highly inflammable; keep it away from fire or heat.

c. Under strong source of light, examine the lens for dirt or finger prints.

Separating Cemented Elements:

Place a sheet of asbestos on the low power electric stove. Put a black paper on the asbestos plate and then keep the lenses to be separated. Cover the lenses with bell jar or card box. When the lens is hot enough between 80^{0}C-120^{0}C, gently press the lens element with a rubber tip tool or with a wooden stick.

Re-cementing:

The process is similar to separating. One should clean the lenses and put on the hot plate with a surface to be cemented together facing up-ward. When elements are hot enough put a little balsam on the surfaces to be joined together. Use lens-centering instrument to check and center the optical elements.

Collimation in Binocular Microscope:

1. Set the microscope.
2. Use a large flat object and focus it accurately.
3. Observe whether or not the eyepiece and diaphragm combine to make a complete a circle. If it is imperfect or the collimation is improper, then collimate the instrument with the following steps :
   a. If the eyepiece diaphragm test shows that it is due to the objectives, check the screws on the mount.
   b. If the instrument is more than half the diameter out of collimation, it is likely that prism is displaced. Prism cell should be checked properly.

Removal of Parallax:

Parallax is a condition brought about when the reticle of an instrument does not lie in the same plane of the objective lens. It can be removed from optical system by repositioning the objective lens as necessary to have its image in the same plane as that of reticle. Having completed all repairs to your instrument, re-clean all the parts to remove traces of moisture, dirt, metal chips and grease from the surface.

Handling of Optical Components and Instruments:

Handling of optical components while in process or during assembly work is tricky job as the surfaces of the quality optical components are very delicate and sensitive. The workman or user should compare the optical components and instruments with a newly born baby.

Most careful attempts of unskilled hands to clean optics or to repair optical instruments results in many scratches and pits, sometime even chipping of the optical components at the edges. This may also happen with a skilled workman, if he is not careful.

The following defects in optics occur mainly due to bad handling or carelessness:

a. Scratches and pits.

b. Stain marks.

c. Edge chipping.

d. Coating deterioration.

e. Strains.

Scratches and Pits:

Though it is a very tough job to produce absolutely scratch free optics, deep scratches and pits visible with the naked eye are disallowed.

These scratches and pits results when a workman is not careful about cleanliness of his hands, gloves and cleaning clothe. Of course, cleanliness of the working place is also very important. The floor, ceiling, walls, working tables, machines and furniture of the laboratory or workshop should be cleaned frequently, so that no dust particle is present to make a scratch. Scratches are also occurring while cleaning the protective layer such as shellac etc. Because, there may be harder dust particles and the optical surfaces are rubbed for cleaning, scratches occur.

To avoid this, optical components should be kept in water, alcohol for sufficient time, so the pitch, plaster, resin or shellac becomes very soft and hard rubbing is not allowed.

Optical components or instrument when left necked for some time, may collect dust on them and an attempt to clean them with a piece of cotton (some times handkerchief) spoils the surface and after a few repeated attempts the surface becomes hazy.

In these cases, first of all, the dust from the surface should be blown off with a syringe or blower and the it should be brushed with a soft camel hair brush and then with a soft cloth (cleaned with Teepol liquid soap) moistened with alcohol or acetone.

Stains:

Optical glass in general is sensitive to atmospheric corrosion, especially to moisture and water vapor and also reacts with protecting layers. A polymer is formed on the glass surface, which appears as a stain. By touching with uncleaned bare hands, optics may get stained as the sweat of fingertips and hands reacts with glass.

Glass surfaces spotted with stain marks are not allowed in quality optics as from these points growth of fungus starts. To avoid stain marks, optical components should not be exposed to water, water vapor or moisture.

Fungal growth on the optical components in the tropics has been a problem for many years and there is no evidence that any of the thin films are different to the mycelia attacking the glass. Most fungal damage arises during storage in humidity. Silica gel bag can reduce the attack in humidity to a limited extent.

For cleaning optical components, one can use methylated spirit, alcohol, turpentine oil, acetone, xyline and teepol along with distilled water. One should use clean soft cloth, pegwood, and fine tissue papers for clueing optical components.

Coating deterioration:

The robustness and life span of anti reflection coating and front surface mirrors largely depends upon the quality of the cleaning optics and the order of vacuum and the rate of evaporation. If the cleaning is not sufficient and the surface is not absolutely grease free the coating deteriorates and blister will take place within a very short time. For cleaning front surface mirrors, only soft brushes should be used.

Strains:

Care should be taken while mounting and assembling of the optical components, so that the optical components in mechanical cell do not get stained. The performance of an optical system becomes very poor if the optics gets stained. As the material and labour required for optical components are very costly, proper attention must be given during all stages of manufacturing, repairing and assembly work as well as handling so as to minimize the rejection and cost. Only by careful handling, the life span of optical instrument will increase.

Setting up the microscope:

a. Place the microscope near a large window.

b. Focus the 10X (16mm) objective in the usual way using a well stained slide.

c. Remove the eyepiece and inspect the back lens of objective.

d. If fitted, the sub-stage condenser should be racked up and down until a fair sharp image of the condenser iris diaphragm can be seen at the back lens of the objective, and (when the diaphragm is fully opened), the back lens can evenly be filled with light. With a simple instrument this step can be omitted, use the sub-stage disc diaphragm in an attempt to control glare.

e. Replace the eyepiece. A reasonably good image should be seen and minor adjustments of the iris diaphragm can be made to reduce glare.

Obviously with daylight the source can not be actually focused on the object. However, it can be helpful to hold a pointed article150-200mm from the mirror and to focus this in the field of view. This often ensures fairly good illumination of the back lens. Because the source is almost unlimited size, the exact position of the mirror is not critical. The imaging of the glazing bars in the field of view can often be avoided by tilting the mirror slightly or by placing the microscope closer to the window.

In summary, while daylight provides a very convenient and useful source giving adequate illumination when 'contrast' specimens are used, the more readily controllable artificial external source are generally to be preferred.

Setting up with an Abbe-condenser:

The procedure for setting up a microscope fitted with Abbe-condenser is in principle similar to that adopted earlier, except that the illumination is now provided by an optically designed condenser.

CONDENSER

Abbe Condenser

N.A. - 1.25

F.L. - 10 mm

Variable Focus Condenser

Aplantic Condenser

Optically corrected for Spherical Aberration

Achromatic Condenser

Corrected for both Spherical & Chromatic Aberrations)

N.A. - 1. 4

It is recommended for research & colour photomicrography.

Any sub-stage condenser should have screws for adjustment.

N.A. of Condenser ≥ N.A. of Objective.

HUYGEN EYE-PIECE

$$\frac{\text{F.L of Field lens}}{\text{F.L of Eye lens}} = 1.5 - 3.0,\ d = \frac{f_f + f_e}{2}$$

RAMSDEN EYE-PIECE

F.L. of field lens = F.L. of eye lens, d = 2/3 F

Advantages over Huygen eyepiece:

a. Better correction for spherical aberration.

b. Eye relief is greater.

c. It can have independent cross wires.

KELLNER EYE-PIECE

$F_f = F_e$, d = 2/3 F

ORTHOSCOPIC EYE-PIECE

a. Wide Field.

b. High Magnification.

c. Eye Relief is about 20 mm.

d. Free from distortion.

e. Petzvel curve is less.

   i.e. 20% less than Ramsden Eye-piece.

4

UV-VISIBLE SPECTROPHOTOMETER

Electromagnetic radiation is an excellent tool for separating the chemical constituents. It consists of electric, magnetic field right angles to each other alternating at 10^{16} times/sec and is propogated in space as a train of waves (see Fig. 1). It has a range beginning from Y-rays to microwaves. Table – I depicts the range of electromagnetic spectrum.

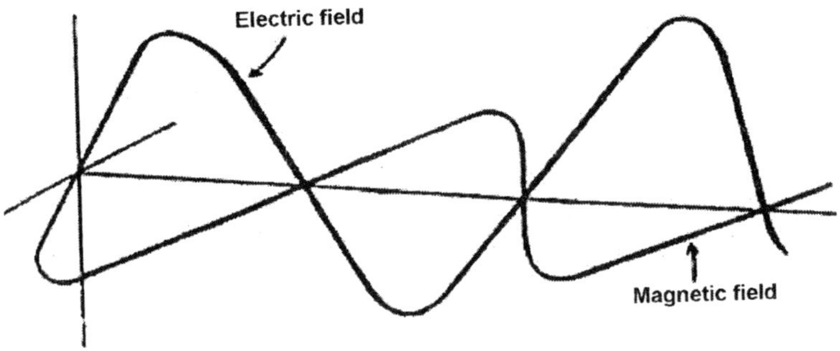

Fig. 1

Different regions of electromagnetic spectrum are used to separate different substances (chemical substances). We shall

Table - I: The Electromagnetic Spectrum

Y-rays	0.01	-	0.1 A°
X-rays	1	-	10 A°
Vacuum Ultraviolet	10	-	1800 A°
Ultra Violet (UV)	180	-	400 nM
Visible	400	-	700 nM
Near Infrared (NIR)	0.7	-	15 μ
Far Infrared (FIR)	15	-	200 μ
Microwaves	0.1	-	1 cm

confine to ultraviolet to near visible spectrum to separate chemical constituents. The basis of uv-visible spectrum is the excitation of electrons in atoms and molecules of a given chemical sample to higher energy levels as a result of absorption of radiation of proper frequency (ν). The frequency absorbed is related to energy difference (ΔE) between two states by the relation $\Delta E = hf = hc/\lambda$, where f, c, λ, n are frequency, velocity of light, and wavelength of light and Plank constant respectively. Mostly, the absorption in uv-visible is due to electronic transition in molecules. The absorption is always due to $\sigma \rightarrow \sigma^*$, $\pi \rightarrow \pi^*$, $\eta - \pi^*$, charged and ligand field-transitions.

Most of the NIR absorptions are due to overtones and combinations of fundamentals normally observed in mid-IR. One advantage of NIR range lies in use of water as a solvent because of transparancy. This advantage allows one to dissolve solute in water and some organics in the region 2000-2500 nM resulting into a "finger print".

The basic relation between absorption of radiation and concentration of the absorption species is governed by Beer's Law viz.

$I = I_0 e^{-abc}$ . . . . (1) where

lo = intensity of incident radiation

a = absorption coefficient

b = path length

c = concentration of absorption species

Thus, in general log lo/l = abc = absorbance = optical density. Absorbance is directly proportional to concentration (c) for a given path length at any given wavelength (λ). If lo/l = 100% transmission (T) then,

Absorbance = log 100% (T) / % T = 2-log (% T). The simplest way of using absorption method is to measure absorbance for standard solutions where concentration is known & then compare these results with absorbance for unknown sample. There is no direct method to find absorption. It is always found by measuring transmission before and after absorption, the previous transmission being adjusted to 100% value. The instrument by which these observations are taken is referred as spectrophotometer.

Instrumentation:

The spectrophotometer consists of following components viz.

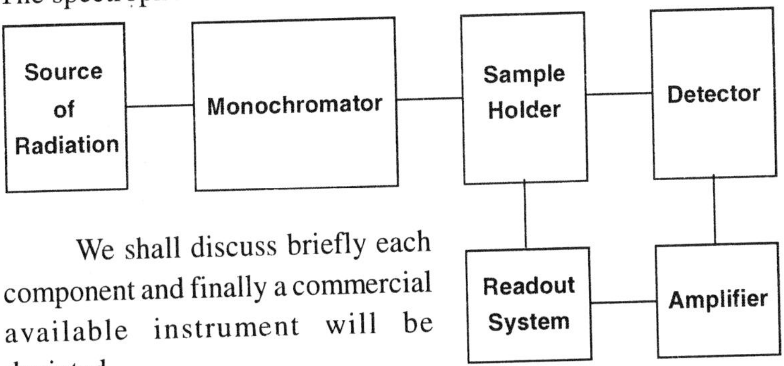

We shall discuss briefly each component and finally a commercial available instrument will be depicted.

Radiation Sources:

The choice of source radiation depends upon emission of number of wavelength and should have uniform intensity over entire range of wavelengths. Such a source, of course, can not be realized in practice and intensity of real source varies with the wavelength. Two types of radiation source are in vogue viz. a) thermal sources b) electric discharge sources.

a) *Thermal Sources:*

Tungsten filament lamp is the most widely used thermal source in the visible region. Energy output of this source depends upon the temperature & is given by Wien's displacement law $\lambda maxT = 0.29$ cm °K. The maximum energy output at $\lambda = 500$ nM leads source temperature to 6000°K however the melting point of tungsten is 3600°K there by limiting operating temperatures to 3000°K. Similarly at $\lambda = 960$ nM (i.e. in NIR) the source temperature is 3000°K yielding maximum emission hence only a small portion of output is available in visible region. The unwanted infrared is removed by inserting a heat absorbing filter between lamp & sample holder.

b) *Electric Discharge Tubes:*

The useable output in uv range is not available with thermal sources of radiation. This has necessitated to develop radiation sources in uv. The simplest uv source is hydrogen electric discharge tube. This works on the principle of excitation of atoms / molecules due to inelastic collisions between bombarded electron and gas molecules. The H_2 discharge tube is the most commonly used as uv source operating at 40V dc at the pressure 0.2-0.5 torr. The continuous spectrum of H2 extends from 165 nM to 400 nM attached with a fused silica window. The major drawback of H_2 discharge tube is due to small energy output with $20^0 < \lambda < 375$ nM. This led to the search of new source viz deuterium. The deuterium lamp while more costly 3-4 times but intense has longer life. The life time is usually decided by number of useable hours and wattage.

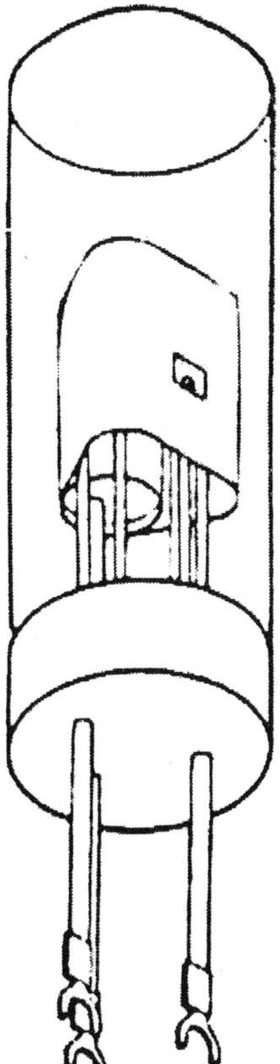

Deuterium Lamp

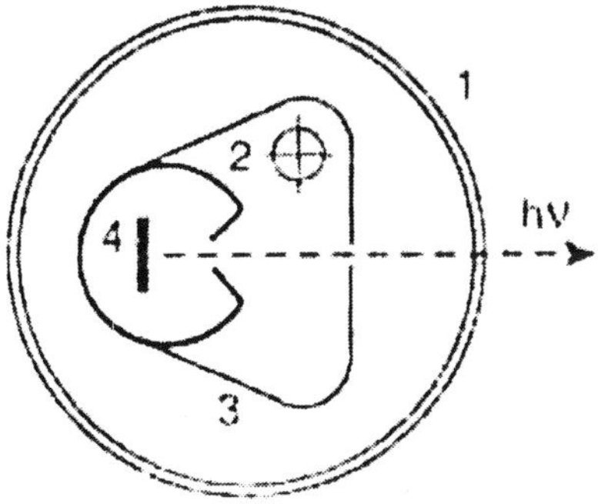

Lamp, seen above
1 - Silica envelope
2 - Filament (cathode)
3 - Metallic screen
4 - Anode

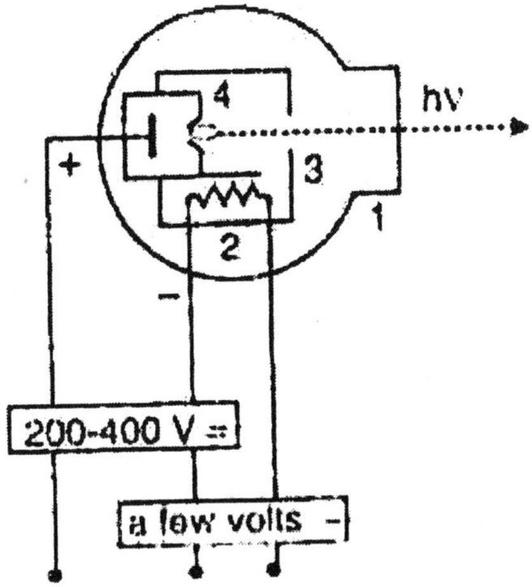

Connections

Fig. 2

The mercury arc is not useful for continuous spectral studies but useful whenever the wavelength calibration of monochromator is out. It has more than 35 atomic lines between $127 < \lambda < 700$ nM with $\lambda = 546.1$ nM being the strongest line. Even Hg are is not used there days and has been replaced by the –Ne laser of $\lambda = 632.8$ nM for calibration and alignment.

The most important aspect of source is stability. The final current (I) in the photodetector is proportional to the nth power of source voltage (v) i.e. $i \propto V^{\eta}$ with $3 < n < 4$. Hence a small charge in voltage can affect the reproducibility of results. This is achieved by using constant voltage transformers and regulators.

Monochromators:

The function of the monochromator is to disperse the radiation available by selecting a proper wavelength (λ) to be incident on the sample. It should maintain constant energy at all wavelength when there is no sample in the instrument.

At present in market two types of monochromators are available based upon their used in single beam or double beam.

In a single beam instrument, the wavelength disperse in a littrow mode. The grating operates on the principle of diffraction in which light is cut off by several slits (width << 1 mm) drawn either by a mechanical engine or by holographic technique resulting into breaking of radiation into several wavelengths (see Fig. 3).

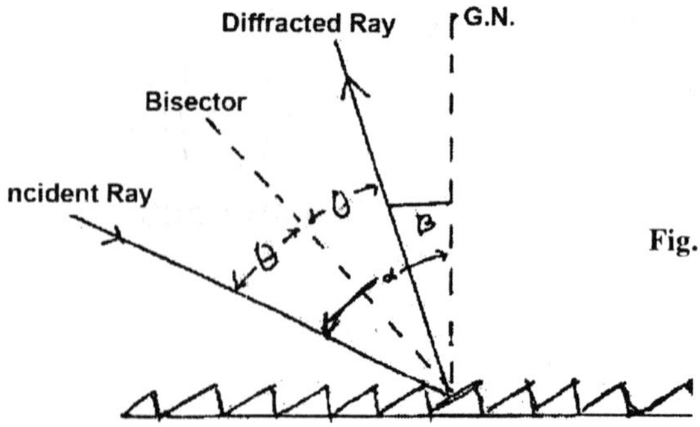

Fig. 3

$\angle$ BOC = $\propto - \beta = 2\theta$. The angle of incidence (α) and angle of diffraction (β) are related by the equation $n\lambda = d(\sin\alpha \pm \sin\beta)$ where n, d are number of orders and grating constant respectively. Each grating is recognised by its grating constant (d) viz. number of lines drawn per num and is generally between $600 < d < 1800$ per mm. The monochromator for single beam instrument operates with the setting $\alpha = \beta$ yielding. $\eta\lambda = 2d \sin\alpha = 2d \sin\beta$ (see Fig. 4) and is called as Littrow setting.

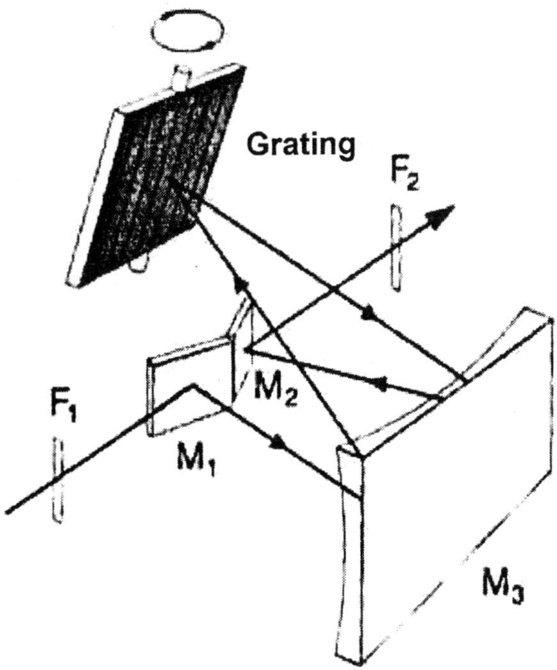

Fig. 4

$nd\lambda$	=	$2d\cos\beta d\beta$
$d\beta/d\lambda$	=	$n/2d\cos\beta$
$dx/d\lambda$	=	$F\, d\beta/d\lambda$
$d\lambda/dx$	=	$2d\cos\beta/nf$

Usually n = 1 can achieved by blazing the grating. As the value of cosβ doesn't change appreciably, one put cos β = 1 & d = 1/600 mm, f = 300 mm, dλ/dx = 2d/f = 2/6000 x 300 = 10 nM/ mm.

The scanning of light beam is accomplished by cam or micrometer screw and with $0 < \beta < 23^0 <$ from uv to visiible.

Reciprocal linear dispersion i.e. change in wavelength per mm is 10 nM/mm. This therefore defines the limit of operation. By keeping slitwidth 1 mm, the available resolution is ≈ 10 nM.

The monochromator used in double beam instrument is of Czerny-Turner type (see Fig. 5).

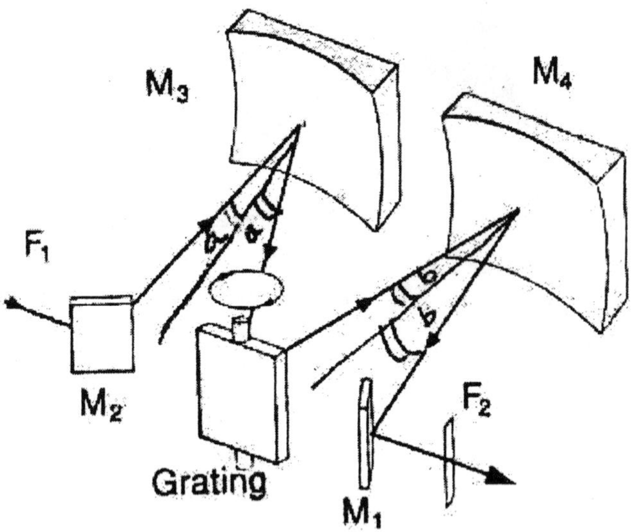

Fig. 5 Czerny-Turner design:

The beam is steered by through a slit and mirror on concave mirror (whose focus generally 250 mm determines the size of instrument) & falls on reflecting grating. After diffraction, the beam falls on second focussing mirror and spectrum is seen on exit slit. In this arrangement, the focus of concave mirror decides the reciprocal linear dispersion and spectral band pass. To obtain higher deflection, the reflectivity of mirror is of the order 99% and use of two mirrors cancels the aberration introduced during steering of beam. The greatest advantage of system lies in zero chromatic aberration and whatever spherical aberration introduced can be checked by suitable stops. The best focus (f) condition is obtained when grating to mirror distance is 0.8452 f. To reduce the comatic aberration, the bisector angle (θ) is set to $\theta = a\sqrt{3} = b\sqrt{3}$ with $5<a$, $b<10^0$. The choice of a, b given θ using

$\beta = \alpha + 2\theta$ in grating equation gives

$$\sin \alpha + \sin (\alpha + 2\theta) = n\lambda/d$$

$$\sin (\alpha + \theta) = n\lambda/2d\cos\theta$$

Thus, the choice of θ gives α & β for a given λ. Like wise reciprocal linear dispersion is given by.

$$d (\sin \alpha \pm \sin \beta) = n\lambda \text{ (keeping } \alpha = \text{constant)}$$

$$\cos \beta \, d \beta = n \, d \lambda$$

$$d\beta / d\lambda = n / d\cos \beta$$

$$\text{Linear dispersion} = dx/d\lambda = f \, d\beta/d\lambda = nf/d\cos\beta$$

$$\text{RLD} = d\lambda/dx = d\cos\beta/nf$$

$$d = 1/12000 \text{ cm}$$

$$f = 250 \text{ mm} \ \& \ 0 < \beta < 23^0$$

$$d\lambda/dx = 3.3 \text{ nM/mm}$$

SBW = Spectral bandwidth = RLD x slitwidth = 3.3 nM/mm z 1 mm = 3.3 nM & 0.3 nM for 0.1 mm slit width. Thus, a better resolution is possible in Czerny – Turner mount with the best possible optical fidelity. However, this resolution is coupled with a penalty in loss of energy output due to the diffraction and requires compensation by choice of suitable detector.

Detectors:

The criteria for selection of photo sensitive detector in uv-visible is based upon sensitivity, response time, spectral response, stability and amenability of out-put to amplification. These choices have led to following devices.

1. *Photo tube:*

A typical phototube consists of concave shape photocathode (of potassium/sodium) with its inner surface coated light sensitive layer. When a radiation is incident on photocathode, photoelectrons are emitted, provided photon energy exceeds a certain threshold. The number of photoelectrons available per unit time is directly proportional to radiant power. Hence, photoelectric detector is radiant power to electric current transducer. Then electrons are collected by the anode and causing a change potential across resister R. The photo current available are in the region of 10 pA which can be amplified. This detector works reasonably well within $400 < \lambda < 700$ nM.

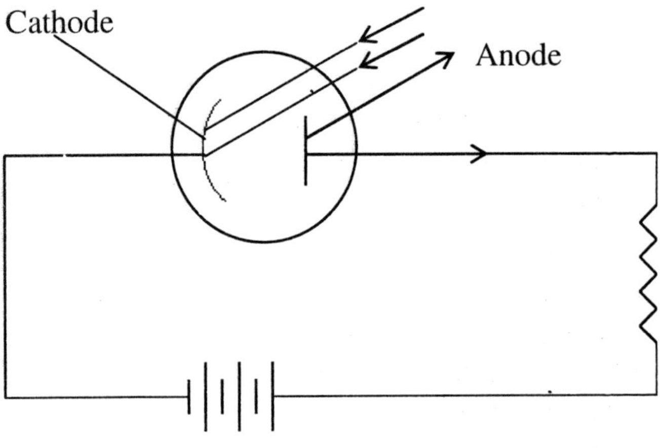

Fig. 6

2. *Photomultiplier Tubes:*

These have a fast response with a net amplification of the order of 10^6 within one tube by the emission of secondary electrons. The final gain depends upon interstage dyanode voltages & therefore a stable power supply is the most important requirement. The superiority of this tube over ordinary phototube lies in detecting a low level signal which is not amenable by the phototube lies in detecting a low level signal which is not amenable by the phototube. The lower limit is set by dark current and noise. The typical response time is 10^{-9} sec. The output is a linear function of incident intensity over a fairly wide range. These tubes need shielding from stray light and magnetifield due to extreme sensitivity.

Cuvette / Sample Holder:

The light after selection from monochromator passes through sample holder. The sample holder for double beam instrument made up of quartz to incorporate the measurement in uv and visible together. They are generally cylindrical in shape for allowing light beam to pass through opposite faces, from solutions. In single beam instrument, the choice is limited to pyrex test tube marked upto which solution is kept in the path of light.

Display / Readout System:

Most of the spectrophotometers (single, double beam) employ either analog meters / digital meters / PC monitor or recorder. However, there is distinct disadvantage in using analog meters as they themselves eat a part of absorbance signal available resulting into loss of information. The accuracy of direct reading meters is limited to 1% FSD. This limits the accuracy to two digits in absorbance. To over come this defect in earlier versions a null balance method was used. In this method one generates a signal using potentiometer & battery equivalent to absorbance signal &

observe null in galvanometer. Linearity of slide wire having accuracy upto 0.01% ensured that the signal of interest is not lost.

The null technique has now been replaced by digital voltmeter. The advantage of digital technique lies in instant measurement, historical trend, no loss of signal and accuracy upto 5 digits being possible. Modern spectrophotometer therefore use digital meter as an essential ingradient for displaying information.

Even digital meter now have been replaced by writting suitable programmes in assembly language by PC. PC now controls the choice of slitwidth, RLD, SBW, concentration etc. More & more sophistication have been introduced as instrumentation progresses.

Typical Instrument Design:

There are two basic designs viz single beam & double beam spectrophotometers.

1. *Single beam Spectrophotometer:*

Fig. 7 shows the layout of the system. An 8V/32W, tungster lamp is energised by constant power supply. It passes through field lens, aperture & talk on grating where diffraction / breaking of radiation take place. The mixture it several wavelength is further controlled by stop before talking on exit slit, cuvette & photo tube. The grating mount is pivoted on steel bulb & carries an arm linked kinematically to sine bar mode to the lead screw or car. As the wavelength drum moves in backward / forward direction a typical wavelength appears on exit slit & passes through cuvette.

As the instrument measures the absorption coefficient (a), the minimum number of steps are (i) with no radiation falling on detector (shutter close). The meter (digital / analog) is adjusted to read zero % transmission (ii) with the solvent in measuring position, the shutter is opened & amplifier gain is adjusted to read 100%

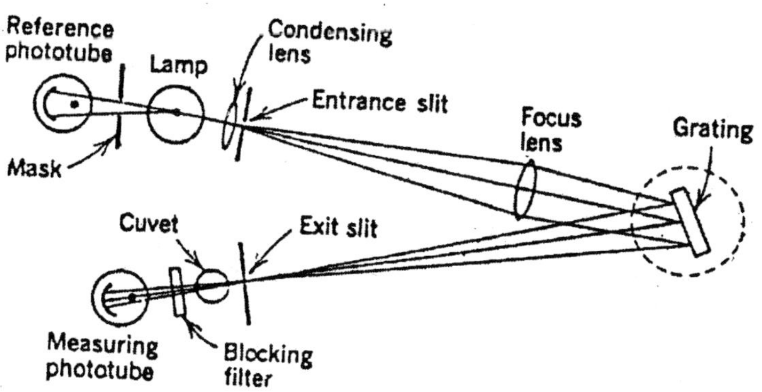

Fig. 7

transmission (iii) with the sample solution in measuring mode, a typical transmission is noted. By adjusting each time solvent is 100% transmission mode one can obtain an unknown concentration by plotting absorbance again concentration.

2. *Double beam:*

Fig. 8 shows the typical commercial system with tungsten / denterium lamp for analysis. The beam from the lamp is steered by set of mirrors in Czerny - Turner setup. At exit slit, the beam is divided into two parts, one passing through solvent & other through sample. To distinguish both the beams property the sample beam is chopped appearing as a pube output while solvent beam as a dc output at the defector. The minimum no. of step required for operating a double beam system are (i) with nothing in the path of sample & solvent, the instrument zero is adjusted, (ii) with solvent in both arms 100% transmission is adjusted (iii) with solvent in one arm & solute in other absorbance is noted. This arrangement has advantage that the effect of source fluctuation is cancelled. By carrying out observations for number of concentrations, one records absorbances from which unknown concentration can be found out.

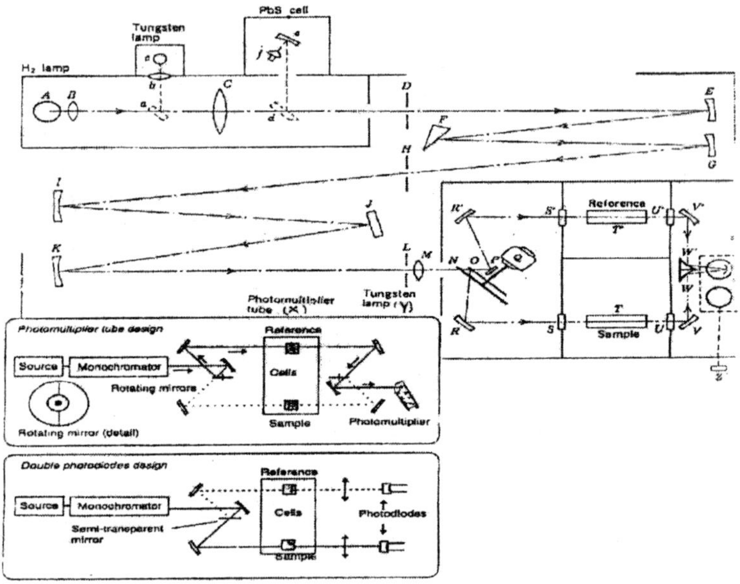

Fig. 8

Applications:

Modern instrumental analysis demands the use of sophisticated uv-visible instrument which addresses the choice of slit width, number of components in mixture, display of SBW, RLD & finding out unknown concentration using graph of absorbance against concentration. The simplest experiment to do in lab is to analyse binary mixture of $KMno_4$ & $K_2Cr_2O_7$. To learn the use of uv-visible instrument, one prepares 5 x 10^{-4} M & 2.5 x 10^{-4} M concentrations of $KMno_4$ & also of 2-5 x 10^{-4}M of $K_2Cr_2O_{7\ \&\ 0.5\ M}$ in H_2SO4. A spectrophotometer sensitive between λ = 340nM to 700nM is needed. First, measure the abosrbance of three Standard Solutions at 500nM & work downward & for $KMno_4$, start at 600nM & work down. One notices that single beam instrument does not offer much as far absorbance is concerned. By repeatation, of this exercise with double beam yields spectacular results. One is unable to find out fine structure between 520 > λ < 580nM in $KMno_4$ solution if slit width is closed to 1mm. The mapping of spectra is meaningful with fine structure details only when slit width is close to 0.1 mm or less than that.

To analyse unknown, choose λ = 350 nM at which $K_2Cr_2O_7$ has maximum absorption. Find also absorbance of $KMno_4$ solutions at this wavelength. Choose another wavelength (λ) 550nM at which $KMno_4$ has maximum & measure the absorbance of $KMno_4$ & $K_2Cr_2O_7$ solutions at this wavelength.

Now take absorbance measurement for unknown at each of wavelengths chosen. Calculate the molar concentration of Mn & Cr in the solution. Note that the calculation is quite easy as dichromate dies not absorb at 550nM. One can use absorbance at λ = 550nM to compute permagnet concentration, then calculate absorbance at λ = 350nM, subtract this absorbance from that you measured & use the difference to compute concentration of dichromate.

In using this method to determine Cr the acidity is important because H_2^+ ion repress the hydrolysis of dichromate:

$$Cr_2O_7^{2-} + H_2O = 2CrO_4^{2-} + 2H^+$$

But H^+ ion also combine with dichromate to form $HCrO_4^-$ & $Cr_3O_7^{2-}$. Acidity therefore will affect the absorption spectrum. This is just one application.

In general, spectrophotometric analysis are very rapid & do not destroy the sample, the absorption spectra are featureless & are of broad band type. The absorption spectrum of a mixture is equivalent to absorption spectrum of individual components. It is very useful to determine dissociation constants of acids & bases; steric configuration and study of free radicals & ion.

REFERENCES:

1. Modern Chemical Analysis & Instrumentation H.F. Watt, J. Reyes, Marcel Dekker Inc. Newyork (1973)
2. Instrumental Analysis, CK. Mann, T.J. Viuckera, W.M. Gulick Harper & Rav Publishers (1974)
3. Modern Optical Method of Analysis, E.D. Olsen, McGraw Hill Book Co. (1975)
4. Instrumental Method of Analysis, H.H. Willard, L.L. Merrittand J.A. Dean, Affiliated East-west Press Pvt. Ltd. (1971)
5. Instrumental Methods of Chemical Analysis, G.W. E wing, McGraw Hill Co. (1969).

5

APPLICATION OF UV-VISIBLE SPECTROPHOTOMETRY

Colour spectrometers are photometer instruments used in Spectrophotometry to measure the intensity or transmitted light as function of wavelength or colour. There are many applications for spectrophotometers, such as measuring the amount of light absorbed by a medium the light is passing through. Spectrophotometers are also used to measure the amount of light which have been reflected by an object, these are called reflectance spectrophotometers.

There are two major classes of measurements performed by spectrophotometers; these are called single beam and double beam. Single beam spectrophotometers measure the change in light intensity of a single light path through a medium. A double beam spectrophotometer compares the light intensity of two separate light paths and determines a ratio.

Colour spectrophotometers are available as hand size, remote mounted, desktop or as a full integrated system unit.

Photometry is a very versatile technique and has diverse applications throughout industry including, aerospace, material manufacturing, pharmaceutical, pulp or paper, building materials, food, glass, paint or coating and plastic industries.

QUALITATIVE ANALYSIS:

Visible and ultraviolet spectra can be used to identify classes of compounds in both the pure state and in biological preparations.

QUANTITATIVE ANALYSIS:

For determining an unknown concentration of a given species. Any system, which is responsible for imparting colour to the compound, is called chromophore. e.g. Most of the nitro compounds are yellow in colour. Thus, nitro group is a chromophore, which imparts yellow colour.

MODERN DEFINITION:

The chromophore is defined as any isolated covalently bound group that shows a characteristic absorption in UV or visible region. e.g. carbonyls, acids, esters, nitrile group of ethylenic or acetylenic group

Chromophores are of two types:

i. Chromophores containing p electrons and involved in $\pi \rightarrow \pi^*$ transitions. e.g. acetylenes and ethelynes.

ii. Chromophores containing both p and n electrons and involved in $\pi \rightarrow \pi^*$ and $n \rightarrow \pi^*$ transitions. e.g. carbonyls, nitriles and azo compounds.

Auxochromes are groups which by themselves do not act as chromophores but whose presence brings about a shift of the absorption band towards the red end of the spectrum (longer wavelength).

Auxochrome is thus also known as a colour enhancer. Examples are -OH, -OR, -NH2, -NHR, -NR2, -SH etc.

Auxochrome exerts its effects by virtue of its ability to extend the conjugation of a chromophore by sharing of the non-bonding electrons. This results in a new chromophore, which has a different absorption maximum and probably an enhanced extinction coefficient.

In many instances the absorption and absorbance change either due to interaction with an auxochrome or due to change in solvent.

Four such absorption and intensity shifts are known.

Bathochromic shift : This shift is due to the presence of an auxochrome by virtue of which the absorption maxima shifts towards higher wavelengths (known as 'red shift'). Sometimes decreasing polarity of the solvent may also cause this type of shift.

Hypsochromic shift : This shift is due to removal of conjugation and a change in the polarity of the solvent due to which the absorption is shifted towards shorter wavelengths (also known as 'blue shift').

Hyperchromic effect : The effect signifies an increase in the intensity of the l max., or a change in the ε to a higher value at the same l max.

Hypochromic effect : It is caused due to introduction of groups which cause distortion in the geometry of absorbing molecules (intensity of λ max is lowered).

UV absorption spectroscopy can characterize those types of compounds, which absorb UV radiation. These compounds are with unbounded electrons (*n* electrons) or those with the conjugated double – beam system (π electrons) such as aromatic compounds. Identification is done by comparing the absorption spectrum with the spectra of known compounds from the references.

UV absorption spectroscopy is one of the best methods for detecting impurities in organic compounds.

The bands due to impurities are very intense. e.g. 0.05% impurity has an ε value of 2000. Therefore, such an impurity can be detected in a transparent major component. The organic compounds can be classified into saturated compounds having little absorption and unsaturated compounds having strong absorption bands. Common impurity in cyclohexane is benzene. Its presence can be easily detected by its absorption at 255 nm.

If Adiponitrile and hexamethylenediamine –the starting materials in nylon manufacture are not pure, then the quality of the nylon obtained is poor. Traces of unsaturated and aromatic impurities can be detected because the starting materials are transparent in the near UV region.

If a compound is being purified, the process should be continued till band due to impurity disappears completely. If the impurity does not absorb whereas major component does in UV region, the purification procedure must be continued until the value of ε becomes a maximum value and corresponds to the value of emax of the 100% pure compound.

The amount of impurity can be determined by using the formula

$$\log I_0 / I_t = \varepsilon c l$$

APPLICATIONS OF SPECTROSCOPY TO ORGANIC COMPOUNDS :

Detection of conjugation:

Conjugated compounds is the major area where a UV spectrum can give a lot of information about structure, which is difficult to obtain by other methods.

It helps to show the relationships between different groups, particularly with respect to conjugation.

The conjugation may be (i) Between two or more carbon – carbon double (or triple) bonds, (ii) Between carbon – carbon and carbon – oxygen double bonds, or (iii)Between double bonds and an aromatic ring.

It can reveal the presence of the aromatic ring itself and the number of locations of substituents attached to the carbon of the conjugated system.

Conjugated polyenes show several UV bands in the >200 nm region. The band at the highest l value has been of great use for structural information.

In general, *cis*-polyenes absorb at longer wavelengths and have lower intensity than *trans*-polyenes. The *s-trans* conformer absorbs at a lower wavelength than the *s-cis* conformer. The *s-cis* conformer shows a band of lower intensity than the *s-trans*.

Carotenoids are a group of widely occurring conjugated polyenes responsible for the colour of carrots (α, β, γ carotenes), tomato (lycopene), etc. The carotenoids show several bands which can be grouped according to the region where they occur, e.g. $\lambda 1$ bands in the visible, $\lambda 2$ bands in the near and $\lambda 3$ in the far UV region. There are three intense bands in $\lambda 1$ region and these are responsible for the colour of the carotenoid. β-carotene has UV bands at λmax 425 nm, 451 nm, and 482 nm, which give carrots the yellow colour. The carotenoids stimulated several systematic studies of conjugated compounds of different types. The presence of hetero- atom and'/ or a charge in the conjugated chain leads to appearance of colour with a smaller number of double bonds. e.g. cyanine dyes.

The dienes are classified into four groups according to their band position: Acyclic (220nm); Semicyclic (230nm); Cyclic (homoannular) (256nm); and Bicyclic (heterannular) (238nm). The UV bands of acyclic polyenes are useful in elucidating the conformation. The relative amounts of *s-cis* and *s-trans* conformers of a diene in the equilibrium mixture can be calculated from its UV band.

Conjugated ene-carbonyl compounds: Conjugated enals, enones, enoic acids and their derivatives show two characteristic bands, a strong one at about 220 nm and a weak one at about 300nm. UV spectroscopy can be used as a sensitive probe for delocalisation, i.e. resonance, which is difficult to detect by other methods (deviation from co-planarity reduces resonance and lowers λ max. The intensity of the bands is also increased by the resonance.

Aromatic compounds with polar substituents: Polar substituents, whether electron withdrawing or electron releasing, effect a red shift in the two accessible bands of the benzene ring (λmax 200nm and λmax 260 nm bands). The shifts are much larger than those induced by alkyl groups (in some cases 200nm band may be shifted beyond 250 nm).

Basically, the UV spectra of these compounds may be expected to give information about the changes in the electronic energy of the ring MOs brought about by substituents due to resonance, inductive and steric effects of substituents. The ratio of the wavelengths of the two bands i.e. λ_{200}nm/ λ_{260} nm is constant for all the substituents and is found to be 1.2. Ideally the spectra of compounds should be recorded as dilute solutions in a non-polar solvent (e.g. hexane) which is to be taken as standard solvent.

Detection of geometrical Isomers: In case of geometrically isomeric compounds, the trans isomers exhibit λ max at slightly longer wavelengths and have larger extinction coefficients than the *cis*-isomers. Stilbenes (C_6H_5-CH = CH-C_6H_5), the *trans*- isomer show λ max = 294 nm (ε =24,000) while the *cis*-isomer has λmax = 278 nm (ε =9,350).

The geometrical isomers -*cis* and *trans* – of transition complexes can be easily distinguished from their visible spectra e.g. the cis-isomer of $[Co(en)_2F_2]NO_3$ is violet whereas the trans isomer is green.

Detection of Functional Groups:

It is possible to detect the presence of certain functional groups with the help of UV spectrum. Even the absence of any absorption > 200 nm is of some utility since it shows the absence of conjugation, carbonyl group, and benzene rings in the compounds. In UV absorption spectroscopy, the absorption curve is influenced by the whole molecule as well as by the particular group that contains the absorbing electrons. This creates difficulty in identifying the presence of any one particular group.

Since no information can be obtained about the non-chromophoric part of a molecule the UV technique alone is seldom enough for complete structural elucidation of an unknown compound. Other spectral data like IR, NMR, etc. can be utilized in practice along with UV.

Structure of Inorganic Compounds:

Absorption spectra have been widely used to solve many problems in inorganic chemistry. Absorption spectra studies have revealed that deep blue colour of ferric thiocyanate is due to the presence of $FeCNS^{2+}$ ions. The proportions of $FeCNS^{2+}$ ions in various mixtures have been calculated using spectra. The structure of coloured substances formed by ferric chloride with phenolic compounds has been studied.

Absorption Spectra of Biological Macromolecules:

Amino acids such as tyrosine, phenylalanine, tryptophan and histidine show an increase in λ_{max} and extinction if they are shifted to a less polar environment. If the absorption spectra of protein changes significantly with changes in polarity of the solvent, the amino acids showing changes in λ_{max} and extinction must be on the surface of the protein. If the λ_{max} and extinction of any amino acid is higher in a protein than the λ_{max} and extinction in the free form, then that amino acid must be surrounded by non-polar amino acids i.e. 'buried'. λ_{max} and extinction always increase for an amino acid if a titration group (SH of cysteine, OH of tyrosine, imidazole of histidine, etc.) is charged. Therefore, upon change in pH: (a) If change in absorption characteristics as a function of pH shows that the ionizable group has a pK comparable to pK in its free state, then the concerned amino acid is on the surface of the protein. (b) If change in absorption characteristics shows a pK widely different from that in the free state, the particular amino acid must be surrounded by strongly polar groups. (c) If no spectra change is observed even at the pH at which titration would normally have taken place (if the AAs was free) then the concerned AA must be surrounded by non-polar groups. As the stacking of purines and pyrimidine increases, i. e., when their ring systems become more parallel and nearer to each other, the extinction of the solution decreases.

Structural Analysis of Macromolecules:

Determination of double stranded DNA:

DNA absorbs at 260 nm. This absorbance increases when DNA solution is heated. This indicates that temperature induces unstacking of DNA. Some very important properties of DNA were discovered from this simple assay. It was noted that the tepm. at which OD 280 increase was higher for DNA rich in guanine-cytosine content as compared to DNA, which had prevalence of adenine-thymine. This indicated that guanine-cytosine pair was hydrogen bonded more tightly than adenine-thymine pair.

Studies based on solvent perturbation of nucleic acid:

Spectral characteristic of mononucleotides are different in a solvent which is 50% D_2O as compared to a solvent 100% H_2O. This change in spectral characteristic, however, does not occur in base pairs. This simple difference allows us to determine how many nucleotides in a nucleic acid are base-paired. Consequently, this assay is very useful in determining the structure of tRNAs.

STRUCTURAL STUDIES OF PROTEINS:

Spectrophotometric titrations of proteins:

Side chains of many amino acids contain ionizable groups which are available for titration. Determination of pK values for proton dissociation from these ionizable groups often provides a good indication about the position of these amino acids in the protein.

Let us assume that a protein has 5 residues each of tyrosine and histidine. An assay of spectral characteristics of tyrosine in this protein shows that tyrosine is absorbing at λ_{max} 300nm (normal λ_{max} being 295) and that its extinction also is significantly higher. One can conclude that tyrosine residues in the protein must be existing in a strongly non-polar environment. If we compare spectral characteristics of histidine in the protein by placing the protein in 100% water and in 20% glycerol + 80% water, tremendous differences in the spectral characteristics of histidine between the two solutions are found. One can conclude that histidine residues exist on the surface of this protein group, which is available for titration. Determination of pK values for proton dissociation from these ionizable groups often provides a good indication about the position of these amino acids in the protein.

Denaturation studies of protein:

Denaturation involves large-scale unfolding of the protein which can bring to the surface chromophores, which were buried when the protein was in native conformation. Such an exposition on the surface brings about the change in the absorbance due to these chromophore groups. Such spectral changes when followed can give valuable data about the denaturation behavior of a given protein. One can study the denaturation behavior of proteins by varying factors such as ionic strength or the temp. instead of the pH.

Binding of small molecules to proteins:

Whenever the substrate or the competitive inhibitor binds to the protein, it affects the polarity of the region or makes certain amino acid residues, hitherto accessible, unavailable. In doing so, it might quite frequently cause some spectral changes, which may be measured. If these spectral changes are compared to the results obtained with other studies such as the solvent perturbation or the spectrophotometric titration, quite a bit of information about the structure of the active site might be obtained.

Molecular weight determination:

If a compound forms a derivative with a reagent which has characteristic absorption in another wavelength region, the molar absorptivity ε of the derivative is almost the same as that of the reagent. However, the OD is different for compounds of different mol. wt. The mol. wt. of the compound can then be calculated on the basis of its absorption data. Molecular wt of amine picrates, sugars, and many aldehyde and ketone compounds have been determined by this method. The method has an accuracy of $\pm$ 2%. Mol. wts. of only small molecules may be determined by this method.

Other physicochemical studies:

UV-visible spectrophotometry has also been used to study physicochemical phenomena such as heats of formation of molecular addition compounds and complexes in solutions, hydration equilibrium of carbonyl compounds, association constants of weak acids and bases in organic solvents, tautomeric equilibria involving acid base systems, protein-dye interactions, chlorophyll-protein complexes, vitamin A aldehyde-protein complex, association of cyanine dyes, determination of reaction rates, determination of labile intermediates, and dissociation constants of acids and bases.

Examples of structure deduction by UV-Vis spectra:

The earliest example where considerable information could be deduced from a UV spectrum was that of mycomycin, an antibiotic having the formula $C_{13}H_{10}O_2$.

A more recent example where UV spectra were helpful is that of structure of prostaglandins (PG).

Another application is the determination of the position of methyl group in the structure of azelain, a flavonol glycoside isolated from rhododendron

References:

1. Organic Spectroscopy by V.R.Dani
2. Biophysical Chemistry – Principles and Techniques by Upadhyay, Upadhyay, Nath
3. Instrumental methods of analysis Analytical Chemistry by G.R.Chatwal and S.K.Anand.
4. UV-visible Spectroscopy by C. N. R. Rao.
5. Principles and Techniques of Practical Biochemistry Ed. B. L. Williams and K. Wilson

6

SPECTROFLUORIMETER

Any fluorescent molecule has two characteristic spectra, the excitation spectrum and the emission spectrum. The excitation

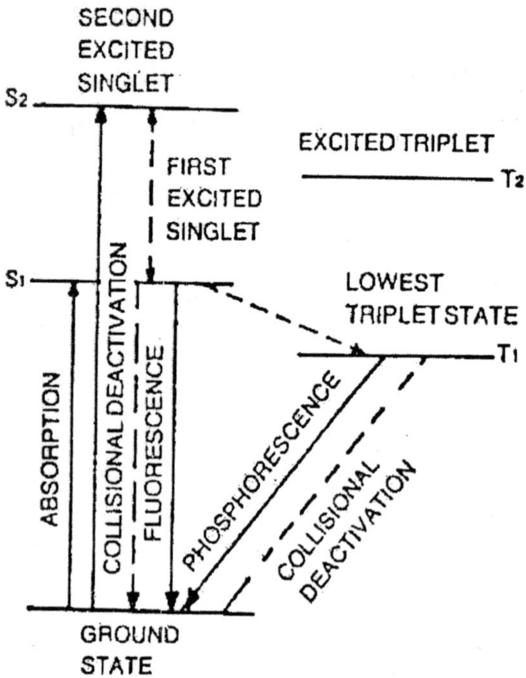

Fig. 1 Principle of fluorescence and phosphorescence

spectrum shows the relative efficiency of different wavelengths of exciting radiation to cause fluorescence, whereas the emission spectrum would indicate the relative intensity of radiation emitted at various wavelengths. Normally, the shape of the excitation spectrum should be identical to that of the absorption spectrum of the molecule, and independent of the wavelength at which fluorescence is measured. However, due to instrumental errors, this is seldom the case. Also, the shape of the emission spectrum is independent of the wavelength of exciting radiation. If the exciting radiation is at a wavelength different from the wavelength of the absorption peak, there will be less absorption of radiant energy, and consequently less energy will be emitted.

It may be noted that *luminescence* is the generic name used to describe all forms of light emission other than that arising from elevated temperature.

Photoluminescence relates to the emission of light through absorption of ultraviolet or visible energy. Photoluminescence can be further divided into :

Fluorescence, which is the immediate release (10^{-8}s) of absorbed light energy as opposed to phosphorescence, which is the delayed released (10^{-6} - 10^{2}s) of absorbed light energy.

Chemiluminescence's is the emission of light energy caused by chemical reactions.

Bioluminescence refers to the light emission through the use of enzymes in living systems.

Relationship between concentration and cluorescence intensity:

The total fluorescence intensity is equal to the rate of light absorption multiplied by the quantum efficiency of fluorescence η, that is

$$F = \eta (P_0 - P) \qquad ...(1)$$

where P_0 is the power of the beam incident upon the solution and P is its power after traversing a length b of the medium. ...(2)

In order to relate F to the concentration c of the fluorescing particle, we can apply Beer's law. In such a case, the fraction of light transmitted is

$$\frac{P}{Po} = e^{-rbc}$$

where τ is the molar absorptivity of the fluorescent molecules and *rbc* is its absorbance A. ...(3)

$$1 - \frac{P}{Po} = 1 - e^{-rbc}$$

$$(P_o - P) = P_o(1 - e^{-rbc}) \quad \text{....(4)}$$

submitting Eq. (3) in Eq. (1), we get

$$F = \eta P_o(1 - e^{-rbc})$$

For very dilute solutions in which A (τbc) <0.05 and only a small fraction of light is absorbed, the exponential term can be expanded, and Eq. (4) reduces to

$$F = K'.\eta.P_o(2.3\tau bc) \text{ or } F = K.c_M$$

This equation shows that for very dilute solutions, a plot of the fluorescent power of a solution versus concentration of the emitting particles would be linear. However, at higher concentrations linearity is lost and the curve bends downwards as the concentration increases.

MEASUREMENT OF FLUORESCENCE:

Fluorescence measurements are carried out in instruments called fluorometers or fluorimeters. The various components of these instruments are similar to those in photometers. These are

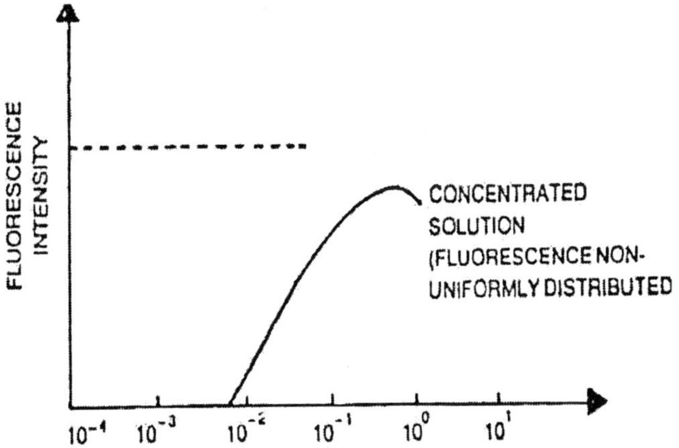

Fig. 2 Plot between concentration and fluorescence intensity

analogous to photometers, as they too make use of filters to restrict the wavelengths of the excitation and emission beams. Fluorescence measuring instruments making use of monochromators like spectrophotometers are called spectrofluorimeters. These are of two types; in one type, a filter is employed to limit the excitation radiation and grating or prism monochromator to isolate a peak of the fluorescent emission spectrum. The other type of instruments are equipped with two monochromators. One of the monochromators restricts the excitation radiation to a narrow band, whereas the other permits the isolation of a particular fluorescent wavelenghts. The latter type are the true spectrofluorimeters.

Single-beam filter fluorimeter:

Fig.4 shows a schematic diagram of a single-beam filter fluorimeter. The source of light is a high pressure mercury discharge lamp, with glass or fused silica envelope. Selection of the exciting wavelength is made by inserting a primary filter in the incident beam. This enables to isolate one of the principal lines at 365, 405, 436, 546 or 579 nm and to have intense line spectrum with

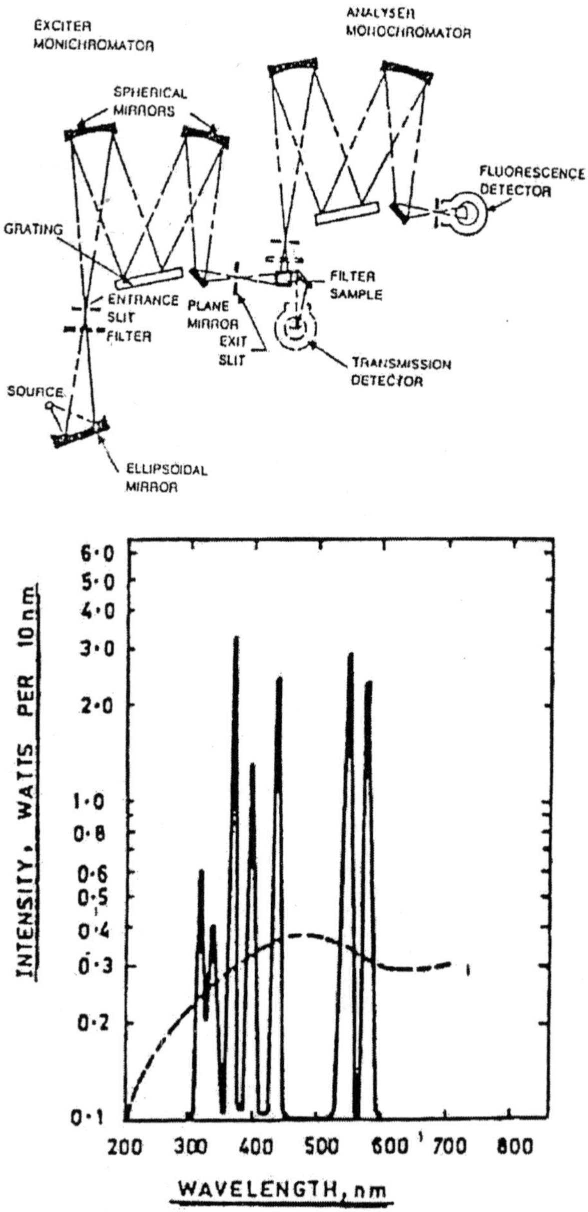

Fig. 4 Schematic diagram of the optical components of typical fluorimeter

good spectral purity. Low pressure lamps, equipped with a silica envelope can produce intense radiation at 254 nm.

Sources:

For luminescence measurements, a continuous source of radiation is preferable to a line source as it can be employed for a large number of analyses. Also, it would be ideal to have a source of uniform intensity over the entire range of wavelengths of interest. These requirements, of course, cannot be met in practice. Intensity of a real source varies with wavelength. The most widely used radiation sources in luminescence spectrometry are xenon, xenon-mercury, or mercury are lamps. Spectral characteristics of xenon and mercury arc lamps are shown in. The xenon spectrum is continuous over the entire ultraviolet region. The mercury arc produces a discrete spectrum or a line spectrum. If a compound under investigation has an excitation wavelength that corresponds to one of the mercury lines, a significantly greater sensitivity results, results due to the high intensity of mercury lines.

Ratio fluorimeter:

Fig. 7a is illustrates the double-beam principle employed in some double-beam filter fluorometers (also called ratio fluorometers).

This instrument makes use of a specially designed mercury-vapour lamp (Fig. 7b) with two anodes on opposite sides of a central structure which combines a symmetrical cathode with a light shield. The lamp operates on A.C. supply connected in such a way that the two anodes receive the discharge, and hence produce radiation, on alternate half- cycles of the exciting voltage. This has the same effect as a rotating shutter, so that the sample and standard receive identical radiation at a frequency of supply voltage. The two beams pass through primary filters, and the fluorescence from the sample and standard converge through a common secondary filter into a single photomultiplier, which sees a series of pulses (Fig. 7c). The electronic circuit sorts out these pulses and the magnitude of the reference pulses is used to monitor the dynode voltages on the photomultiplier so as to maintain a constant reference level. Then the sample pulse produces a meter deflection which can be converted to read directly the concentration of the analyzed species.

Double-beam filter fluorimeter:

Double-beam instruments are direct reading type and are generally preferred because of this obvious advantage. In these instruments, the cirucit is so arranged that the current from the reference detector opposes that generated by the measuring photocell. The reading on the calibrated scale, at which the two currents neutralise each other directly gives the fluorescence reading.

Fig.8 shows a snematic diagram of a double-beam fluorimeter. A mercury lamp is used as a source of radiation. A collimated beam is passed through the primary filter, which then falls on a cuvette containing the sample. The measuring photocell is mounted at right angles to the excitation beam. Fluorescent radiation passes through secondary filters, which remove scattered ultraviolet radiation, but pass visible light.

A part of the excitation beam is passed through a reduction plate for reading the intensity of the reference beam, in order that its power be of the same order of magnitude as the weak fluorescent beam. The attenuated reference beam is reflected on to the surface of a reference photocell, mounted on a rotating table. By adjusting the angle of the photocell, the amount of radiation falling on the photocell, and thus the current output, can be adjusted.

The outputs of the reference and the measuring photocells are compared and a sensitive galvanometer is used to check the null-point. The circuit is arranged, so that the current from the reference cell opposes that generated by the measuring photocell, which responds to fluorescent radiation. In this arrangement, the concentration C is given by

$$C = K\frac{R_{AB}}{R_{AC}}$$

where R_{AC} is the total resistance. The constant K is independent of P_o. Quite often, two photocells, connected in parallel, are used to measure the weak fluorescent radiation. This arrangement increases the sensitivity of the instrument. Fig. 9 shows the schematics of a ratio fluorimeter.

Spectrofluorimeters:

Spectrofluorimeters are true fluorescence spectrometers, which normally make use of two monochromatros, one to supply selectively the excitation radiation and the other to isolate and analyse the fluorescence emission. The dual monochromator system thus allows to determine and selectively utilise the peaks of excitation and fluorescence wavelength. The spectrum of the fluorescence emitted by the sample can be studied at any frequency of exciting light. Also, the variation of the intensity of fluorescence with the frequency of the exciting light used can be determined.

Fig. 10 shows a schematic of the optical system used in a spectro-fluorimeter. The source of light is a 150W high pressure xenon arc lamp. The ellipsoidal mirror collects radiation from this lamp and focusses an enlarged image of the arc upon the entrance slit of excitation monochromator, completely filling the f/3.5 mirrors.

Monochromatic radiation of specific wavelength is selected by angular positioning of the grating. A desired band-pass is achieved by the selection of appropriate interchangeable slits for the entrance and exit positions of the monochromator. The radiant energy emerging from the exit slit of the excitation monochromator activates specific molecules within the sample, resulting in fluorescent emission. The emitted radiation is viewed by the analysing monochromator, which permits only characteristic sample emission to reach the detector, blocking all undesired spectral regions. Schematics of two commercial models are shown in Figs. 11 and 12.

Baired Atomic Model SF 100E spectrofluorimeter (Fig. 13) employs a unique optical system, comprised of four grating monochromators; two are used in tandem for dispersing excitation energy and two used for observation of fluorescent spectra. This double-grating system in conjunction with folded optics offers a significant advantage in the reduciton of physical dimensions. Each monochromator incorporates a 600 line/nm plane reflection grating. Wavelength control is provided by means of a cam, which may be operated manually or automatically. The calibrated operating range of each pair of monochromators is 220 to 700 nm. Wavelength settings are indicated by a scale, which is calibrated in 2 nm increments. The spectral widths of the entrance and exit slits to each pair of monochromators are each independently variable, in steps of 2,8 and 32 nm.

The excitation source is a specially selected 150W dc xenon arc lamp, which gives a very stable, high intensity light output in the UV, visible and infrared regions. An off-axis ellipsoidal mirror forms an enlarged image of the source arc at the entrance slit of the excitation monochromator. The lamp can be readily focussed and laterally adjusted.

The detector used is a photomultiplier, which is supplied with a stabilised power supply. The detector signal is amplified in an operational amplifier.

The optical bridge principle:

The PMT is mounted inside a rotating cylindrical interrupter, with two sets of light slots. The upper slots allow light to pass alternately to the PMT from the rear calibrated light path and the combination of the sample and forward light path. The lower slots interrupt the light path from the reference beam, which in turn generates the reference signal. This circuit arrangement cancels out variations in line voltage, light source and photomultiplier sensitivity (Fig. 14).

The PMT produces an ac signal at about 400 Hz, that is proportional to the light unbalance. This signal is amplified and fed as signal to the phase-sensitive detector.

The reference signal is generated by a lamp with special glass filter around it, which passes only infrared light and directs it on to red-sensitive phototube. The reference lamp and phototube generates an ac signal. This signal is amplified and is given as reference to the phase detector, its phase depending upon the position of the light interrupter. The phase detector generates a dc signal proportional to the signal received, which is applied to the chopper, where the dc signal is converted to ac.

Microprocessor-based spectrofluorimeter

Iwata et al. (1986) described the details of a microprocessor-based spectrofluorometer (Fig.15). The instrument takes advantage of the microprocessor in both instrument control and data manipulation originating in the data station unit (DSU). The microprocessor enables to have a variable spectral bandwidth in steps from 1.5 to 20 nm, wavelength scanning speeds selectable in steps from 1 to 1000 nm/min, a software-controlled shutter that closes the aperture of the excitation monochromator and an auto-zero function.

Sensitivity improvement in the instrument is achieved by : (i) Using holographic gratings of 1800 grooves/mm. The stray light of this optical system is less than 3.5% at 220 nm excitation wavelength and 5-nm spectral bandwidth. (ii) Rotating the slit image of the monochromator formed on the sample cell by 90^0, in which the observed volume of the sample illumination is enlarged by the slit's length-to-width ratio, resulting in higher emission intensity and an increase in sensitivity.

A dynode-feedback technique is employed to compensate for the characteristics of the light source.

DETECTORS:

Single channel detectors:

Phototubes

Photomultiplier Tubes (PMT):

Blue sensitive : 200 - 600 nm

(Maximum response - 300 - 500 nm)

Red sensitive : > 600 nm

Noise reduction : by cooling

Analog detectors : Current generated intensity or Current pulses generated by individual incident photons are counted.

Multichannel detectors:

Simultaneous acquisition of emission or total luminescence spectra with increased range of application to

Real time experiments

Kinetic measurements

On-line detection for chromatography and other flow systems (e.g FIA)

Ability to acquire complete spectral information essentially instantaneously which facilitates the analysis by dramatically reducing time

Types :

Diode arrays

Vidicons

Silicon-intensified Target (SIT) Vidicons

Charge-Injection Devices (CID) / Charge-Coupled Devices (CCD) (Detailed description of detectors is given under "Spectrophotometers")

Single photon counting instruments:

Measurements at very low light levels

Maximum signal / noise performance

Double monochromator arrangement to minimize stray light

Cooled PMT housing to minimize detector noise

Ratiometric detection to minimize effect of variation in source output .

PMT detects a portion of excitation beam that is directed to the detector by a beam splitter placed between excitation monochromator and the sample

Appropriate blank in the reference beam : absorption measurements can also be made

Depiction of single photon counting. The signal is detected by the PMT, emerging as a pulse which is then amplified. If the magnitude of the amplified pulse exceeds a certain threshold, it is passed through the discriminator and counted as a signal. Smaller pulses due to noise and dark current are much more likely to be rejected, thereby increasing signal-to-noise.

Instruments with special capabilities:

1. *Extended spectral acquisition:*

Excitation and Emission spectra +

Synchrnous excitation spectra +

Total luminescence spectra

Emission and excitation monochromators

scanned simultaneously and synchronously

Array detectors: reduce time by allowing simultaneous measurement of intensity at many wavelengths

Spectrograph is used to disperse the emission beam and simultaneously detect all wavelengths in a given range.

Two-dimentional array detectors for total luminescence spectra

Rapid scanning instrument:

Exit slits are removed from ex and em monochromators to convert them into polychromatros. Excitations wavelengths are spatially resolved along the vertical axis of the sample cuvet and therefore the detector, and emission wavelengths are spatially resolved along the horizontal axis of the detector.

A silicon-intensified target vidicon serves as the two-dimensional detector.

Advantages: Reduction in analysis time

Improvement in S/N ratio

Ability to perform multiwavelength kinetic studies

Minimization of sample decomposition

2. *Polarization measurements:*

Fluorescence polarization can be measured. Polarizers can be placed in both the excitation and emission beams, between the corresponding monochromator (or filter) and the sample

L format: Single excitation channel

Single emission channel

T format: Single excitation channel

Two emission channels (one for vertically polarized component and the other for horizontal component)

Two emission signals measured ratiometrically to eliminate erros due to polarization that occurs in the excitation monochromator.

3. *Luminescence lifetime measurements*:

Determination of excited state lifetimes

Time-resolved techniques

Pulsed source excitation and direct acquisition of decay curve which is analyzed for expotential decay characteristics of the emitting components.

Range depends on : width and reproducibility of ex. pulses detector response generally limited to several nanoseconds or more

Flashlamp source with high repetition rate and time-correlated single-photon counting (TCSPC) - extend the range of lifetimes into subnanosecond range.

Each pulse generates a start signal at PMT which triggers the voltage ramp of the time-to-amplitude convertor (TAC). The ramp is terminated when a photon emitted from the sample is detected. Therefore, the amplitudes of the output pulses are proportional to the time between start and stop signals, which in turn are related to the luminescence lifetime.

Lasers with high repetition rates and fast PMT detection extend the use of TCSPC well into subnanosecond region.

TCSPC is designed for detection of very low level photon signals.

Pulse-modulation luminescence spectroscopy:

This is frequency-domain alternative to pulse methods for lifetime determinations.

Continuous (lamp or laser) source excitation beam is modulated appropriate frequency (MHz for fluorescence lifetimes; Hz to milliHertz range for phosphorescence lifetimes). Luminescence emission will be phase-shifted by an angle ϕ and demodulated by a factor m relative to excitation beam. Values of ϕ and m depend on the modulation frequency and luminescence lifetime of the sample, which can be independently calculated from ϕ and m.

Depiction of the phase-modulation fluorescence lifetime technique, showing intensity-modulated excitation and emission beams with a.c. amplitudes B and B', respectively, and d.c. intensities A and A'. Lifetimes are determined from phase shift f and from demodulation m, where m = (B'/A')/(B/A).

Frequency domain fluorescence lifetime instrument:

A multiharmonic Fourier transform technique is used to acquire phase and modulation data at multiple frequencies simultaneously. A base frequency generated by radio frequency (RF) electronics is converted into a phase-coherent electrical pulse at the harmonic modulator, which drives the Pockel's cell to convert the output of a cw laser into a pulsed signal containing the base frequency and harmonics. Harmonic generators (HG) modulate the gain of the PMTs at a base frequency that is phase-locked to the pulse excitation fequency and slightly offset from it, for phase sensitive detection of the multiharmonic emission signal.

Practical considerations:

1. ***Environmental effects*** **:**

Competition of de-excitation processes Solvent composition, Temperature, pH, Ionic strength.

2. ***Wavelength calibration / Spectral correction*****:**

Emisison monochromators commonly calibrated with standard sources like Hg arc lamp with number of accurately known emission lines from 253.65 to 809.32 nm.

Excitation monochromators the calibrated using a scattering solution to direct the calibrated excitation line through the emission monochromator to the detector.

Acquired spectra can be corrected for wavelength dependency of source output, monochromator efficiency and detector response by various methods : Use of thermopiles, quantum counters, calibrated phototubes with known spectral response curves, and solutions of standard fluorescent compounds.

3. *Background and interfering signals*:

Common source of background intensity scattered light from particulates, Rayleigh or Raman scattering phenomena Fluorescence and phosphorescence may also be mutually interfering.

Appropriate choice of ex. and em. wavelengths scattered light has effective lifetime of zero : so time-resolved or phase-resolved approaches to minimize the contribution of scattered light to an emission signal.

Background signals can be corrected for by blank substraction. Also, derivative spectroscopy, wavelength modulation techique or time-resolved or phase-resolved techniques can be used to improve the selectivity and reduce background interferences.

4. *Fluorescent measurements in the near infrared:*

Fluorescent dyes that absorb and emit in the NIR region (650-1000 nm) gaining popularity as alternatives to uv-visible dyes as labels and probes. Advantages of working in NIR are : NIR dyes have high molar absorptivities and quantum yields approaching 70% when dyes are absorbed on solid surfaces such as gels. Background noise is much lower in NIR so that lower detection limits can be achieved. Availability of small, inexpensive devices for excitation and detection is added major attraction. Soild state diode lasers are rugged, long-lived sources of relatively high excitation power in NIR. Silicon phtodiode detectors provide highly sensitive detection with faster response than PMTs and very low noise levels.

Most useful NIR dyes:

Polymethine family of dyes:

Carbocyanines

Merocyanines

Metal-containing

phthalocyanines & aphthalocyanines

Xanthene family of dyes:

Fluorescein, hodamine

7

FTIR INSTRUMENTATION AND BASIC CONCEPTS

Optical techniques of analysis are based on the interaction of matter and electromagnetic radiation. Most of these methods are not destructive in the sense that sample is not destroyed and can be used for further investigations. These techniques essentially involve the observation of three types of molecular transitions; electronic, vibrational & rotational. The observation of ultraviolet & visible spectra involves electronic transitions while vibration-rotation transitions for infrared. These boundaries are infact loosely defined & overlap does occur. Spectrophotometric technique basically involves measurement of intensity and wavelength absorbed.

The origin of infrared (IR) spectrum lies in the vibrational degrees of freedom in a molecule. Any two masses coupled by a restoring force can execute simple harmonic motion (SHM), when disturbed from their position. This is how one can explain two atoms joined by a chemical bond. The molecular vibrations are the SHM executed by atoms in a molecule about their mean position in the molecular field that binds them. Barring monoatomic and homopolar molecules all substances absorb IR and no two compounds have identical IR spectrum with the exception of optical isomers. This in effect means that IR absorption spectra of a given compound is its finger print & powerful tool for chemical identification and molecular structure elucidation.

The infrared spectrum (IR) can be classified into three regions (i) the near IR (ii) fundamental IR (iii) far IR. Near infrared spectroscopy ($0.7 < \lambda \leq 2.5$ μM) is used for quantitative analysis of different functional groups & absorption bands are due to overtones and combinations of vibrations. Instruments used in near IR are similar to those of visible region. It is the fundamental region $2.5 < \lambda < 25$ μM which is of paramount importance for obtaining qualitative and quantitative information about various function groups & molecular structure. Two types of instruments have emerged over the years viz. (a) dispersive (b) Fourier Transform Infrared (FTIR). This article describes the basic concepts of FTIR.

FTIR instruments are based upon basic principle of superposition of two or more monochromatic electromagnetic waves described by the equation.

$$y = a_1 \sin (2\pi/\lambda)(vt-x_1) + a_2 \sin 2\pi/\lambda\,(vt-x_2) + \ldots..$$

where, y is the displacement of atoms from mean position, a_1, a_2, v, t, x_1, x_2 are amplitude of first, amplitude of second wave, velocity of wave and distances respectively.

It can be shown that path difference between two waves is $(x_2-x_1).2\pi/\lambda$ = phase difference. Setting $x_2-x_1 = \lambda, 2\lambda, 3\lambda$ leads to constructive interference fringes, while $x_2-x_1 = \lambda/2, \lambda, 3\lambda/2$ .... yields destructive interference fringes. To extract information about wavelength line from such a complex waveform was a challenge till the advent of digital computers. With the advent of fast digital computer, it is now possible to reverse the process of superposition of waves to obtain conventional spectra by a mathematical operation viz. ***Fourier Transform***. This in essence means that FT operation allows one to go from one measurement domain to another. The application of FT to the spectroscopy was limited in early stages for the weak signals obtained from stars. The chemical application of FT spectroscopy was first studied by Fellgett around 1967-1970 and subsequently led to the design of commercial instrument in the region $10<\lambda<400cm^{-1}$

There are inherent advantages of using FT as a process to obtain conventional spectra. In the conventional spectra resolution is dependent on the choice of slit width and narrowing slit width leads to less available energy at the detector consequently S/N ratio decreases. Extracting of useful information about transmittance is done by a process callėd signal averaging. In this process signals are additive and noise being random decreases but with a penalty of large amount of time. FT process has a distinct advantages that resolution being constant over entire domain and all the measurements are taken simultaneously. This means if conventional IR takes 10 min. to record the spectra than FT can replicate 600 measurements. Second advantage is that of precision in wavelength (λ) or wavenumber (σ) there by facilitating comparison of spectra. Thirdly, stray light in FTIR is minimal. Optics of FTIR offers a large energy throughout ($\approx$ 50%) than dispersive optics limited by narrow slit. As a consequence of this large amount of energy is accumulated at the detector resulting into more sensitivity.

Conventional spectroscopy is basically a frequency domain spectroscopy as one records radiant power data against frequency (or against wave number). On the other hand time domain spectroscopy, one records radiant power $p(\nu_1)$ data with time. Fig. 1 illustrates the difference.

The curves are figs. c-d is conventional spectra of two monochromatic sources with frequencies v1 and v2 & curve-e indicates spectrum of a source containing both frequencies. Again curve-a indicates time domain spectra for each of monochromatic sources while curve-b exhibits a periodicity or beat as the two waves go in & out of phase. Similarly time domain spectra of

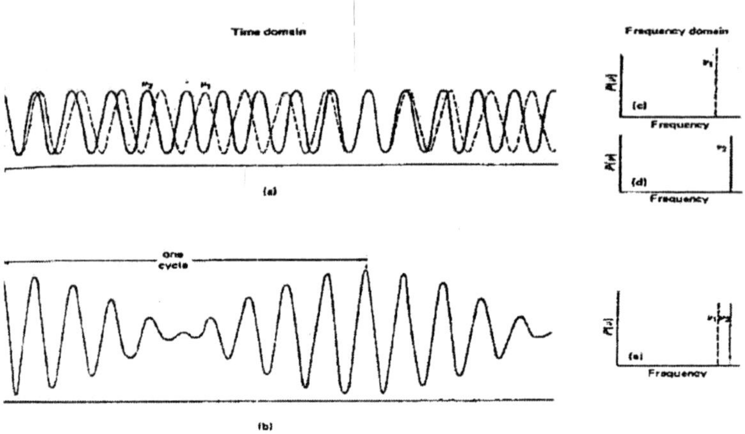

Fig. 1

several wavelengths will be more complex & a full cycle is never realised in time. Further the signal power decreases with time as a consequence of variously closed spaced wavelengths with time & therefore closely spaced wavelengths are more & more out of phase. The time domain in essence contains same information, as does a spectrum in frequency domain. The two can be related as

$$p(t) = k\ (\cos 2\pi\nu_1 t + \cos 2\pi\nu_2 t)$$

where k is a constant. The difference in frequency is generally within ± 10%.

When a large number of spectral lines are involved inter conversion of time & frequency domain spectra becomes mathematically tedious, requiring a high speed computer.

METHOD OF OBTAINING TIME DOMAIN SPECTRA:

Acquisition of time domain spectra requires a transducer (or set of transducers) with a sufficiently rapidly response times. This means 10^{15} Hz<n<10^{7} Hz region of ultraviolet spectroscopy to nuclear magnetic resonance, acquisition of time domain spectra is ruled out. Another, important aspect is that one requires a method of converting (or modulating) high frequency signal to one of measurable frequency. Then only time domain spectra can be recorded. i.e. modulated signal must be proportional to original signal. Different modulation procedures are employed for various wavelengths region of spectrum. Michelson interferometer is extensively used in IR region.

THE MICHELSON INTERFEROMETER:

Michelson interferometer used for recording IR spectra in time domain is slightly modified than conventional one. As shown in Fig. 2, a beam of radiation falls on beam splitter, which transmits approximately 50% of, light & 50% reflected. The twin beams are then reflected from mirrors, one of which is fixed while other moving. The beams then meet at beam splitter with half of each being directed to sample & detector, other two halves being directed back to source.

Once a motion is given moveable power output at detector will fluctuate in a predictable manner. The power output will be maximum when moveable & fixed mirrors are at same distance from beam splitter. With a monochromatic source distance equal to $\lambda/4$ (position B C) will correspond to phase change of $\pi/2$ therefore, power of combine beam will be zero & similarly at (A & D) distance equal to $\lambda/2$ power will be maximum.

δ = Retardation = difference in path of two beams.

$\delta = 2$ (M-F) -- (2)

A plot at detector, δ Vs p (t) is called interferogram.

The interferogram takes the form of cosine function. The power is maximum when $\delta = 0$. Typical infrared scanning interferometer, the mirror is driven at constant velocity V_m cm/sec. Since peak appears at high multiples of 'λ' of incident radiation, the frequency (f) of interferogram is given by.

$f = 2 V_m/\lambda$ --(3)

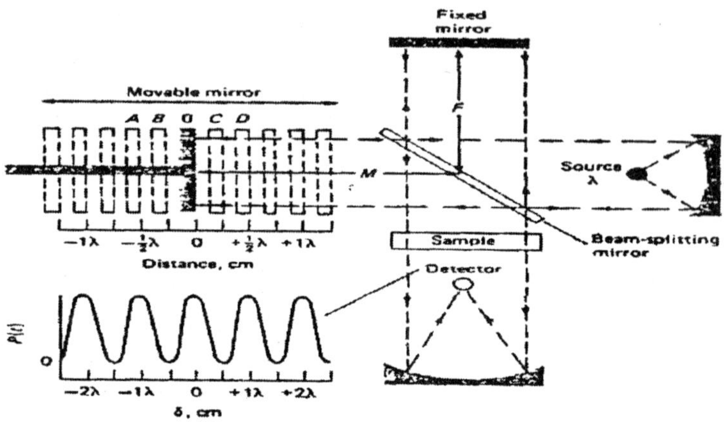

Fig. 2

Factor '2' accounts for the reflection process doubles the effect of retardation. Just to get an idea of frequency of interferogram, we set

$V_m = 0.5$ cm/sec, $\lambda = 2.5$ mm,

16 μm gives, $f_1 = 4000$ Hz, $f_2 = 625$ Hz

This illustrates one important fact that fluctuation in signal power must be fall into audio frequency range. The IR transducer fulfils this conditions hence one can record time domain spectra. Fig. 3 shows time domain spectra along with wave number (σ)

FOURIER TRANSFORMATION OF INTERFEROGRAM:

One can express cosine wave of interferogram

$$P(\delta) = 1/2\ p(\sigma) \cos 2\pi ft \text{ ---------------------------- } (4)$$

when P(σ) is the radiant power of IR beam on inteferometer & P(σ) is the power of interferogram signal. Thus Eq. 4 is a interconnection between frequency domain & time domain. Further

$$P(\sigma) = B(\sigma) \cos 2\pi ft \text{ --------------------------------- } (5)$$

& Substituting Eq. 3 leads to

$$P(\delta) = B(\sigma)\cos(4\pi V_m \sigma t) \text{ ------------------------- (6)}$$

The mirror velocity (V_m) can be written.

$$V_m = \delta/2\,t \text{ --- (7)}$$

This connects interferogram signal with retardation factor (δ) & wave number (δ) of input optical signal. Interferogram in Fig. 3 can be expressed as number of wave numbers leading to

$$P(\delta) = B_1(\sigma)\cos_2 \pi\sigma_1\delta + B_2(\sigma)\cos 2\pi\sigma_2\delta \text{ ------- (8)}$$

and for infinite number of wave numbers (i.e. wavelengths), one has

$$P(\delta) = \int_{\infty}^{\infty} B_n(\sigma)\cos(2\pi\sigma_n\delta)d\delta \text{ ---------------------- (9)}$$

Fourier transform of this integral is given by

$$P(\delta) = \int_{\infty}^{\infty} B_n(\sigma)\cos(2\pi\delta_n\sigma)\,d\sigma \text{ -------------------- (10)}$$

Infrared Fourier transform spectroscopy consists of recording P(δ) against δ & then mathematically transforming this relation to one that gives P(σ) as a function s (spectrum). The Eqns 9-10 assumes that beam contains infinite wave numbers & a mirror drive of infinite length. This is practically impossible further Fourier transform with a computer requires that the detector output be digitized i.e. output must be sampled periodically & stored in digital form. This means sampling intervals $d\delta \rightarrow 0$ should be infinitely small.

RESOLUTION OF FITR SPECTROMETER:

The resolution of FTIR spectrometer is given by,

$$\Delta\sigma = \sigma_1 - \sigma_2 \text{ -- (11)}$$

where σ1, σ2 are the wave numbers for a pair of barely resolvable IR lines. Two lines are resolved if one scan the time

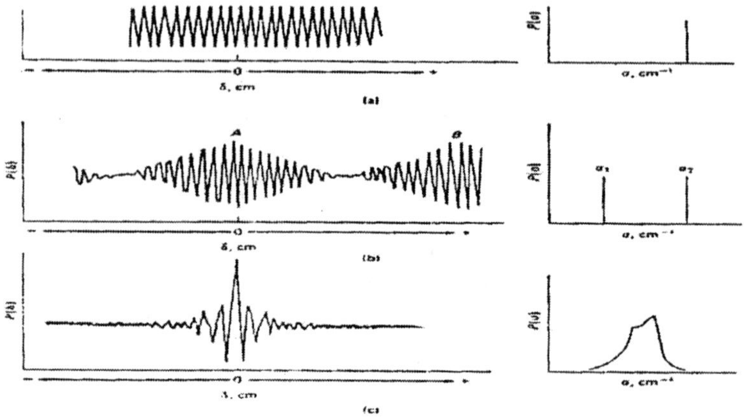

Fig. 3

domain spectra long enough so that one cycle or beat for two lines is completed only then will all information in spectra have been recorded. In fig. 3 would require recording of interferogram from maximum B were two waves meet again in phase. The maximum at B occurs when $\delta\sigma 2$ is larger than $\delta\sigma 1$ i.e.

$$\delta\sigma_2 - \delta\sigma_1 = I$$

$$\sigma_2 - \sigma_1 = 1/\delta \quad \text{---(12)}$$

Suppose one requires a resolution of 0.1 cm^{-1} then one can calculate mirror length by $0.1 = 1/\delta$, $\delta = 10$ cm which means mirror motion required is half of retardation or 5 cm.

Resolution is also influenced by planarity of the mirrors & coplanarity of beam splitter. It is lost if radiation entering the interferometer converges or diverges.

SAMPLING THE INTERFEROGRAM:

Fourier transform of an interferogram can only be computed if one digitize & store radiant power at equal intervals of retardation. This means inteferogram must be broken into resolution elements & power of each of these measured & stored in the memory of computer. Following information theory, the calculation of the minimum number of resolution elements x that will permit reconstruction of spectra from an interferogram without loss of detail is

$$x = 2\,(\sigma_{max} - \sigma_{min}) / \Delta\sigma \quad \text{------------------------------(13)}$$

For example, one wants to reconstruct an IR spectrum from 4000 to 625 cm-1 with a resolution of order 1.5 cm^{-1} then x=2(4000-625)/1.5= 4500

The power for 4500 points would need to be measured, digitized & stored.

INSTRUMENTATION:

A requirement for satisfactory interferograms is that speed of moving mirror be relatively constant & its position exactly known at any instant. The planarity of the mirror must also remain constant during the entire sweep of 10cm or more. The displacement of the mirror in far IR is accomplished by a motor driven screw. The demands are more precise & sophisticated for mid IR & near IR. Here the mirror mount is generally floated on air cushions held within close fitting stainless steel sleeves (see fig. 4). The mirror mount is driven by an electromagnetic coil similar to voice coil in loudspeaker a slowly increasing current in the coil drives the mirror at constant velocity. After reaching the terminus, the mirror is returned rapidly to starting point for next sweep by a rapid reversal of current. The length of travel varies from 2 to 18 cm with speed 0.05cm/sec to 4 cm/sec.

Two additional features of the mirror system are necessary for successful operation in IR regions. The first is the means of sampling the interferogram at precisely spaced intervals. The second is a method for determining exactly the zero retardation point to permit signal averaging. If this point is not known precisely, the signals from repetitive sweeps would not be fully in phase, averaging would tend to degrade rather than improve the signal.

The problem of precise signal sampling & averaging is accomplished by using three interferometers rather than one, with a single mirror mount holding three moveable mirrors. Fig. 4, is one such arrangement. The components for interferometer are identified by subscript 1,2,3 respectively. System I is IR system which provides an interferogram similar curve A in Fig. 5 system 2 is a laser fringe system which provides sampling interval information.

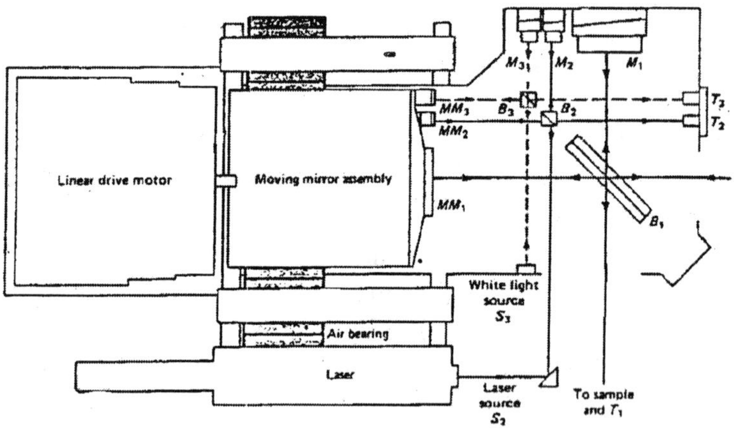

Fig. 4

It consists of He-Ne laser S2, an interferometric system including mirrors MM2 & M2 and a beam splitter B2 & transducer T2. The output from this system is sinusoidal as shown by curve 'C' of Fig. 5. This signal is converted electronically to square wave form shown in D. Sampling begins or terminates at each successive zero crossing. The laser fringe reference system gives a highly reproducible & regularly spaced sampling interval. In many instruments, the laser signal is also employed to control the speed of mirror drive system at constant level.

The third interferometer system employs a tungesten source S3 & transducer T3 sensitive to visible radiation. The mirror system

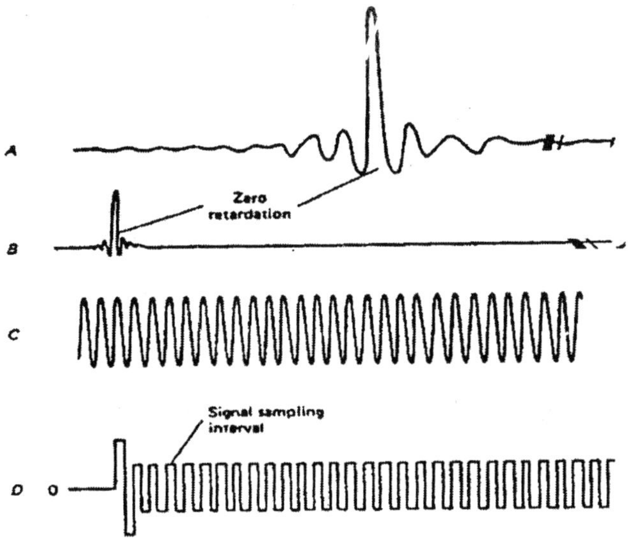

Fig. 5

is fixed to give zero retardation that is displaced to the left from that for analytical signal (see Fig. 5, interferogram B). Because source is polychromatic its power at zero retardation is much larger than any signal before & after that point. Thus, this maximum can be employed to trigger the start of data sampling for each sweep at a highly reproducible point.

BEAM SPLITTERS & SOURCES:

There is constructed & transparent material with refractive indices such that 50% of radiation is reflected. A widely used material for far infrared region is a thin Mylar sandwiched between two plates of a low refractive index solid. Thin films of Ge or Si deposited on CSI, CSBr, NaCl, KBr are satisfactory for mid infrared region.

The traditional IR sources like Globar, Nerst Glower are also used in FTIR instruments at high frequencies. Most generally used source is mercury lamp with silica envelope. It has a distinct advantage over Nerst glower that it radiates energy in longer wavelengths & less at shorter wavelengths. At a frequency below 100 cm^{-1}, the lamp becomes hot & its silica envelope radiates energy. Some worker recommends cooling to improve the stability of arc. Above 60 cm^{-1} tungsten coiled filament is a better substitute than others.

DETECTORS:

In early lays Golay detector was very popular with a high sensitivity over a large range. Only problem is slow response with a chopping frequency 10Hz.

During last 10 years triglycine sulphate pyroelectric detector has been developed & seven times superior to Golay. It has a high chopping frequency 1000 Hz & useful from 2 to 300 μm.

For operation at very low frequencies InSb detector has been proved to be useful on accounts of its high sensitivity with a modulation frequency of 400Hz.

In recent years $Hg_xCd_{1-x}T_e$ has come into use in photo-voltiac mode. It is operated at liquid nitrogen temperature & has a fast response & spectral range 5000 to 400 cm^{-1}.

DYNAMIC RANGE & LINEARITY OF AMPLIFIER:

In normal use, the output signal from interferometer is fed to an analogue/digital converter & digitised equivalent of signal stored for future use or passed on to computer for processing. If system can discriminate 1000 different signal levels from 0 to maximum, the measuring system is said to have a dynamic range of 1000. A minor difficulty in FTIR is that ratio of maximum signal to smallest signal is much greater than for, say a grating spectrometer. Matters are made worse, if power spectrum under investigation consist of broad feature less band, corresponding to the energy emission from black body radiation, together with a few sharp absorption bands. One requires a dynamic range of 10000 to obtain a fair indication of magnitude of ripple. Even this may cause on digitizing error ± 0.5 unit. It is fairly obvious step to increase the amplifier gain as the interferogram signal diminishes, making allowable of course for any change of gains in subsequent computation.

One way to reduce dynamic range is to use double beam system where the gross features of spectrum cancelled out & available dynamic range can be devoted to minor details?

A point not to be overlooked is that the signal amplifier must have high degree of linearity, if an accurate spectrum is to be obtained. If we consider a single interferogram of frequency $\sigma 1$ i.e. continuous cosine wave, any non-linearity in amplifier will lead to distortion of this wave form & harmonics will be introduced. These may eventually produce spurious bands at 2σ, $(3\sigma 1)$ etc, & if spectrum contains one or more sharp bands & the linearity of the amplifier is suspect a search should be made for minor bands in expected positions.

CHIRPING:

The difficulty of large central peak is taken care by putting a flat plate of appreciable dispersion in one optical path & load dispersion in other path. This process leads to chriping of interferogram. Advantage is the reduction of dynamic range.

NOISE: - Three main types of noise are observed.

a. Source Fluctuation

b. Photon Noise

c. Scintillation Noise

a. SOURCE FLUCTUATION:

Source fluctuations are avoided by recording reference & sample interferogram in succession then the ratio-computed spectra. Another method is to record interferogram at high speed & take average of number of spans.

b. PHOTON NOISE:

This arises due to statistical fluctuation in number of photons emitted in unit time by source, which is maintained at constant temperature. It is generally of no importance at longer wavelengths but when a cooled detector is used considerable amount of energy may be received from the parts of interferometer which happen to be within the field of view. Suppose energy per second from a body peaks at 10 μm & wanted signal is weak, under such situation fluctuation in back ground signal is dominant. This is overcome by using refrigerated screen to obstruct the background signal.

c. SCINTILLATION NOISE:

It is due to medium between source & detector & only trouble some in astronomical observations. It is mitigated by proper choice of modulation frequency & also by using double pass interferometer.

SAMPLE ACCOMMODATION:

As FTIR spectrometers are used with an even greater range than dispersive spectrometer, owing to their high sensitivity, the

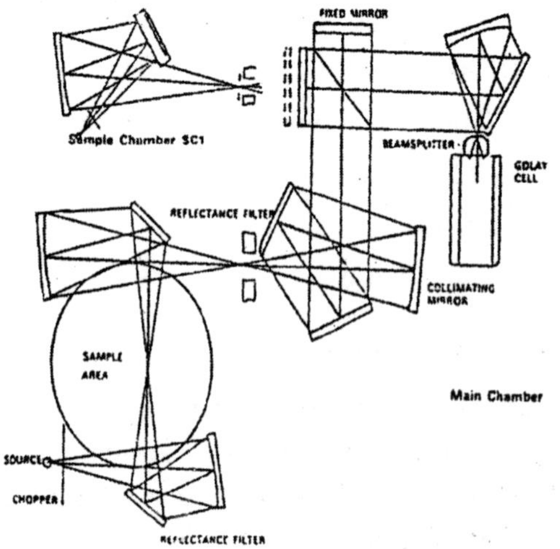

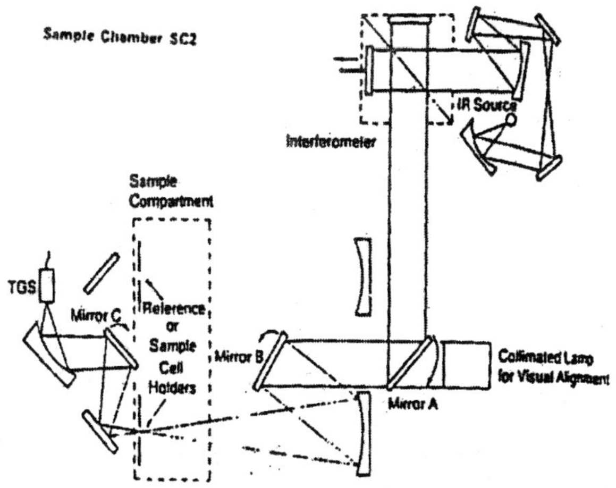

provision of adequate sampling arrangement is quite important. Samples are never kept in front of entrance aperture where it receives maximum intense light. The sample compartment is generally after the interferometer.

8

APPLICATIONS OF FTIR SPECTROSCOPY

Fourier Transform Infrared (FTIR) Spectroscopy is an established analytical technique that identifies compounds by finger print light absorption spectra. The constituents of the sample are revealed through their wavelength dependent absorption bands. FTIR analysis relies on passing a collimated beam of infrared light through sample. The analyte absorbs IR light at wavelengths specific to the functional group present in molecule. Thus each constituent has characteristic IR spectra which can be used to identify the compounds.

Since, it is not possible to know exact amount light absorbed by different constituents of a sample the best option has always been to record transmission of beam before and after absorption, the previous transmission (T) being adjusted to 100% value / standard value. Hence absorbance (A) is directly proportional to concentration (C) given by

$A = 2 - \log (T\%) = abc$ — (1) where a, b, c are absorption coefficient, path length and concentration respectively.

SYSTEM COMPONENTS

A typical FTIR system consists of an IR source, beam splitter, Michelson interferometer, He-Ne laser for beam tracking, detector.

The spectral dispersion in conventional spectrophotometer setup is obtained by a suitable choice of grating. Fourier transform setup uses a principle of superposition of waves in which individual wave form is extracted by a mathematical operation FT from one domain to other using Michelson interferometer setup. The beam from IR source is passed through beam splitter and it falls on a fixed and moving mirror to yield interference fringes. Each component reflected by two mirrors returns to the beam splitter. The moving mirror affects the path of two beams, thus introducing a phase difference. The division of a amplitude beam thus introduces a phase difference. The amplitudes of the waves are combined to give an interferogram, & the resulting encoded beam passes on sample compartment and is detected, by either photon or thermal detector. The entire spectral range is covered by the movement of moving mirror. The detector signal results in an interferogram consisting of complex FT of the spectrum. A specially written computer programme is used to obtain spectrum by carrying out an inverse FT.

The success of FT hinges on displacement of moving mirror with a micrometer screw by a step up motor. To increase precision in movement of moving mirror an electromagnetic coil is also used. The advantage of this system lies in abrupt reversal leading to a starting point for the next sweep.

Another important requirement is precisely spaced retardation intervals for sampling the interferogram. This is absolutely necessary to establish zero retardation point and to facilitate signal averaging. This problem of precision signal sampling and averaging in modern commercial instruments is addressed by use of three moveable mirrors instead of one.

Beam splitter is an essential component for achieving division of amplitude of IR beam from source. The primary requirement of any beam splitter is that it shall transmit maximum of incident IR radiation. Other considerations are refractive index, optical homogenity, cold flow resistance, coefficient of thermal expansion, resistance to gases and solubility in the water. Fuse silica, ZnSe, CsI, KBr, BaF_2 have emerged as material for the beam splitter. Each is transparent in the different region.

There are two classes of detector that are being used for IR region viz. thermal and photodetector. In the thermal detector, the action IR radiation introduces blackening after a millisecond and ceases on its withdrawal. The triglyceryl detector is the common type used in IR absorption studies. The photon detector is a semiconductor and action of IR radiation results into formation of holes and electrons in less than a millisecond. It requires cryogenic cooling. Hg Te is the common detector in this class and is much more sensitive than pyroelectric detector.

Utility of Single Beam & Double Beam Instruments:

The single beam instruments are particularly useful for difference spectroscopy. The most important aspect in such equipment is the source intensity fluctuation resulting into erroneous data. In the double beam instrument the beam from interferometer is alternated between a reference & sample compartment. The absorbed signal is extracted from sample compartment, which is chopped. This arrangement is particularly useful for the studies in mid IR. Resolutions (R) for most of the FTIR instruments lie between $2 < R < 0.01\ cm^{-1}$.

A typical commercial FTIR instrument includes instant display of spectra, updating of fast process such as real time GC-IR spectral acquisition, effortlessly zoom / expansion of any portion of spectrum, ordinate / abscissa axes labels being continuously updated. It also incorporates simultaneous display of as many spectra as desired for the comparison, digital storage facility from which retrieval of the spectra is possible. It can also perform spectral subtractions & base line correction with the rapidity unmatched by conventional IR instruments.

Second type of instruments is tailored to meet specific applications such as microanalysis, GC-IR separation etc. with a facility for spectral search.

Modern FTIR instruments are designed in such a way that it yields data in fraction of seconds. It can perform wide variety of tasks such as subtracting a reference transmission from sample to identify of mixture of a sample & is of crucial importance to quality control applications. Quantitative analysis of multi-component is also carried with software tailored to it. The various types of software are available to perform quantitative analysis. Some of the instruments have the facility for quick change of beam splitter with excellent photometric wave-number accuracy, line shape & sensitive to high-resolution gas phase spectra (eg. NH_3, Co etc.) and superior linearity in the absorbency (A) range $O < A < 3.7$. The linearity in these instruments is a function of quality optics, detector, source, analog, digital amplifiers & data processing.

New generation of FTIR spectrophotometer unit includes treating thermal samples, attenuated total reflectance, circle cells, gas cells of varying path length, photoacoustic cells, beam condenser, flow through cells, vibrational circular dichroism, GC-IR interface, flow cells for HPLC & TGA-EGA-IR facility. It also includes library facilities for GC-IR eluents, those of forensic interest, library for polymer / co-polymers / polymer additives & so on.

General Applications of FTIR:

The maximum utility of FTIR is realized in far-IR region & is particularly useful for the study of inorganic compounds as absorption due to metal-metal bond & metal ligarid bonds below 600 cm^{-1}.

FTIR is an important tool in the study of inorganic solids in far IR region providing information about lattice energies of solids & transition energies of semiconducting materials.

The absorption spectra of molecules composed of light atoms with skeletal bend modes using FTIR yields information on group frequencies. Benzene is a concrete example in this respect.

It is also possible to observe the spectra of Hcl, AsH_3 in far IR region using FTIR. It of course needs purging of water vapour from the setup.

Single FT spectroscopy is useful in mid-IR provided the solutions is dilute & one adopts difference spectroscopy. This difference can't be observed clearly using normal dispersion grating spectrophotometer. The single most utility lie for on the identification of species eluted from GC column. This requires rapid scanning of spectrum & data acquision. FTIR instruments can therefore only do it.

FTIR instruments are not adaptable in emission mode due to poor signal to noise ratio (S/N). It is difficult to identify trace level element when temperature of material under investigation is slightly above the temperature. Even though, some applications have recently emerged, such as identification of microgram quantities in pesticide like DDT. The samples in such applications are prepared in suitable solvent & evaporated on Nacl / KBr plate. The information about spectra is extracted by heating plate.

The proper interpretation of IR spectra leads to knowledge of thickness of films, crystalinity, polymerization, phase change H_2 bonding & kinetic reaction.

Paints, inks, coating can also be analysed by FTIR due to low energy handling & high absorption FTIR is an ideal tool for micro sample, trace gases & nanogram samples & in general for pollution studies.

Another important application is in the area of surface analysis of coatings, catalysis, adhesion, absorption, lubrication, paints and treated surfaces.

The technique also offers a study on monomeric and polymeric species. The crystalinity of polymer can also be determined followed by effect of irradiation damage and mechanical stress.

In semiconductor industry it is used for evaluating Si crystals. Similarly, detection of proteins in H_2O solutions and analysis of haemoglobin can also be carried out by this technique.

The single most use lies in quality assurance environment where speed, accuracy and reliability are of most importance. As the data acquisition is very rapid, it is extremely useful to identify a multicomponent system without operator intervention.

The 5000-3700cm^{-1} region is of particular interest to polymer chemist because of 0% transmission given by main polymer bands.

Other applications include kaolinite (in the region 4800-100cm^{-1} using diffuse reflectance), evaluation of optical response of optical filters, organometallics, metal oxides and transition metal compounds (400-200cm^{-1}).

Using FTIR technique, one can examine chemical reaction or physical changes in progress and characterise reactant and product molecules in time varying chemical reaction (e.g. kinetic FTIR observations of transient species by pulse laser phototysis in millisecond scale).

Semiconductor application includes on-line examination of silicon epitaxial thickness measurement and also of interstitial oxygen.

Highly absorbing aqueous solution pose a serious problem from analysis point of view. It is circumvented by using attenuated total reflectance (ATR) spectroscopy in which effective path-length of IR beam is of the order of 10 μ. ATR is also an effective technique for rubbers, carbon filled polymers, fabrics and o-rings. The acquisition of spectrum is accomplished by placing specimen in intimate contact with a crystal of high refractive index and directing IR beam through it.

Milk samples, triethanolamine are best examined by circular internal reflectance technique as these substances are highly absorbing.

An alternative to KBR is diffuse reflectance spectroscopy. It is useful for pharmaceutical samples and papers. The technique is particularly useful for studying the effect of thermal treatment oil samples before and after treatment.

Laminate polymer material of 10 μ size can not be examined by ATR technique but requires an intimate knowledge of micro-ATR crystals. These micro-ATR crystals provide more reflections per unit area and yield more sensitivity. The application includes spectra of fibre optic coatings, single synthetic fibres and moulding defects.

Incorporation of microscope module in FTIR instrument increases its capability to examine samples of micron size. IR microscope is able to establish fibre standard. Mapping of larger samples, biochemical and semiconductor is also possible. Herbicide concentration in various leaf and plants can also be determined using this technique.

FTIR in-conjunction with process analyser can accomplish analysis of complex mixtures (e.g. aqueous solution of detergent ranging 0.1 to 60% can be determined simultaneously). Other applications include sugar and alcohol in fermentation both and polycomponent solvent mixtures.

Gas cells are available in variety of path lengths. Using multiple pass multicomponent gas analysis of concentration 0.01 to 11 ppm is possible. The application includes environmental measurements, breathing, exhaust gas analysis, gas-phase kinetics, solid and liquid decomposition studies and also extended to evolved gases during thermogravimetric analysis.

A double modulation which incorporates modulation of sample between two states at a frequency well above maximum gives time resolution between 10μs to 1ms is also possible with FTIR. It is useful for obtaining information about chemical kinetics.

Hyphenated technique combining the advantage of GC-FTIR / HPLC-FTIR offers exceptional ease of use, sensitivity & performance while maintaining GC / HPLC integrity & resolution. The complex mixtures can be identified using separation power of GC with specificity & identification power of FTIR spectroscopy. These accessories are designed to work up to 300° C providing the capability to analyse low volatility, high mixture compounds. This interface is particularly designed to analyse small elution volume characteristic of high-resolution capillary column. Excellent sensitivity upto nanogram is possible. Software gives separate identification for GC & IR.

A gold plated light pipe is a common GC - FTIR coupling device. Eluants enter it from chromatographic column through a small diameter stainless steel tubing column that ensures minimum dead volume. It leaves by far end, often to continue to a GC detector viz. flame ionisation detector. In an average light pipe about 25% of the IR beam traverses its length. Whether components can pass through without being band broadened can be ascertain by the response of GC detector to the eluant from the light.

A matrix isolation interface that provides more efficient collection of component has been recently devised. There is no need to correlate flow rate with peak width in this arrangement &

offers low detection limit. Using argon as a matrix gas the column eluate can be spread on a slowly moving cryogenic surface to collect components. Infrared spectra are taken continuously after a standard short time lag.

Usually the IR spectrum is identified by function group followed by a library scanning of related IR spectra, seeking a match to complete the identification of an analyte.

All GC-IR interface include sophisticated chromatographic data processing package, Gram-schmidth reconstruct base line corrections, difference calculations & automatic peak area. The software also includes kinetic applications such as TGA/EGA, photolysis reactions & others.

Poor sensitivity & instability of wave member scale are the main drawbacks of dispersive IR spectrophotometer. Simultaneous participation of all wavelengths in FT operation makes it an ideal choice with HPLC effluents producing IR spectra. This combination allows one to carry out efficiently subtraction IR spectroscopy.

HPLC solvents absorb strongly in mid IR regions leading to inefficiency in spectral curve collection. This can be effectively addressed by automatic blanking of opque spectral areas to eliminate confusion, disallowing solvent spectral contribution, conversion to absorbance & indexing of spectral files.

Thus in essence hypenated technique allows one to have extension of chromatrographic resolution by spectroscopic means yielding enormous amount of information. IR spectral library incorporating spectra of dilute ccl_4 & Cs_2 are ideally suited with many LC/IR flow cell measurements with the advantage that flow cell measurements are taken in a diluted solution in a constant matrix.

Modification of traditional FTIR instrument for environmental chemicals monitoring is a recent application. It employs a Michelson interferometer, He-Ne laser for beam alignment, axicon/retroreflector & detector kept at about 500 m from the source. The monitoring is carried out for volatile organic chemicals (voc) by passing a IR beam through it with amplitude of absorption proportional to concentration. These systems are infact similar to particle counter which sums up total amount of energy that a target chemical absorbs between FTIR & retroreflector. FTIR in itself can not distinguish between a narrow plume or broad diluted plume that contained with in path length. FTIR data is interpreted in-conjunction with meteorological data to discern the potential difference. Concentrations obtained in ppm / ppb are either path averaged or path integrated. In the path averaged concentration are obtained by measured amount of chemical divided by path length. These systems are not typically quantitatively calibrated. The performance of unknown voc is evaluated first by gathering information on target compound. Hue Phan has recently applied these ideas to gasoline samples with oxygenate concentration between 1 to 10% using Midas 2000 FTIR. He also applied this concept to measure voc viz tri chloroethyleve with a relative concentration to 370 ppb to obtain measurable results. Further spectacular advances have also been available in the book "Advances in applied FTIR spectroscopy" edited by M.W. Mackenzie.

More & more studies have been undergoing in different areas using FTIR to gain knowledge about composition of a compound, which will be repository of future generation to come.

9

FLAME PHOTOMETER

PRINCIPLE OF FLAME PHOTOMETRY:

According to the quantum theory, the energy states of an atom or molecule are sharply defined and any change from one state to another therefore, requires a sharply defined quantity of energy. When radiation falls on a material, or the material is supplied with extra energy in some form, some part of the energy is taken up by the material and results in altering the state of the atoms or molecules of which it is composed. The atoms or molecules of the material are promoted to higher energy states. However, the higher energy states are rather unstable. The particles at the higher energy levels tend to lose the extra energy and return to that original level or ground state, either by undergoing a chemical reaction or by dissipating the energy as heat, or by emitting the energy as radiation. If it loses all or part of the energy as radiation, it will emit photons of an energy corresponding to difference between two energy levels. Since the levels are clearly defined for a given atom, the radiation will be emitted at clearly defined frequencies only. The frequencies are shown up as bright lines if the emitted light is dispersed as a spectrum. By measuring the wavelength of the emission, one can find out what atoms are present. Also, by measuring the intensity of the emission, one could compute the concentration of the element.

In short, the principle of flame photometry is based on the fact that if an atom is excited in a flame to a high energy level, it will emit light as it returns to its former energy level. By measuring the amount of light emitted, we can measure the number of atoms excited by the flame.

The method of flame photometric determinations is simple. A solution of the sample to be analysed is prepared. A special sprayer operated by compressed air or oxygen is used to introduce this solution in the form of a fine spray (aerosol) into the flame of a burner operating on some fuel gas, like acetylene or hydrogen. The radiation of the element produced in the flame is separated from the emission of other elements by means of light filters or a monochromator. The intensity of the isolated radiation is measured from the current it produces when it falls on a photocell. The measurement of current is done with the help of a galvanometer, whose readings are proportional to the concentration of the element. After carefully calibrating the galvanometer with solutions of known composition and concentration, it is possible to correlate the intensity of a given spectral line of the unknown sample, with the amount of the same element present in a standard solution.

Flame photometry is characterised by a high degree of constancy and reproducibility. The spectrum of an element as produced in a flame is relatively simple, consisting normally of only a few lines. Identification of the line is simple and spectral interference is less frequent. The most usual application of flame photometry is for the analysis of sodium and potassium in body fluids and these analyses constitute the bulk of the determinations generally performed. However, the method is slowly replacing more troublesome methods for other elements also.

Flame photometry is concerned mostly with atoms. Molecules cannot normally survive the high temperatures employed in flame photometry.

The number of elements to which flame photometric methods can be applied depend mainly on the source temperature developed by the fuel-mixture employed. This is because not all atoms are easily excited in the flame. The atoms of some elements have their energy levels so spaced that a large number of different lines are emitted, while for some others, almost all the light they emit is concentrated in one spectral line. The upper energy levels of atoms of some elements are so high above the ground state that they are very difficult to excite. Also, their emission lines could be of a wavelength, which may not be directly usable. All these factors determine the lowest concentration of atoms which can be detected in the sample and thus varies very widely for different atoms.

Flame photometry offers the following advantages:

- The technique is very rapid. It does not require any chemical preparation except preparing a solution of suitable concentration.
- The method is most useful for analysis of some elements, which are difficult to measure by other methods.
- The technique is most suited to analytical problems, in which a large number of samples of similar types are to be measured.
- The method is quite cheap as it does not require any other expensive reagents.

CONSTRUCTIONAL DETAILS OF FLAME PHOTOMETERS

(a) Emission System:

Consisting of the following:

A flame photometer has three essential parts (Fig. 1)

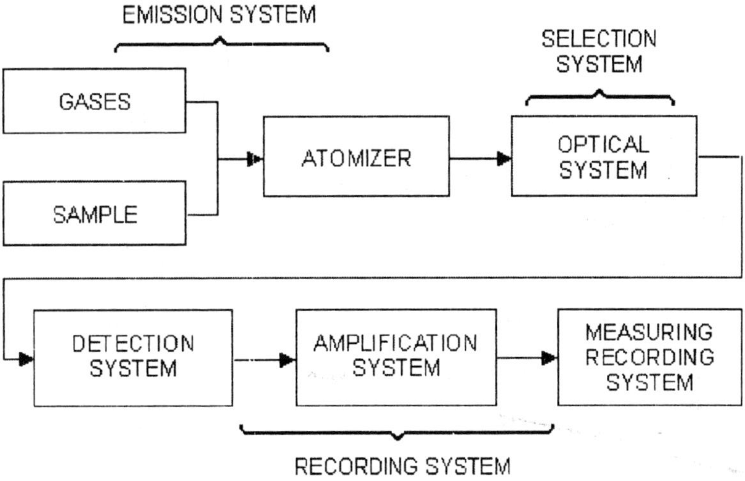

Fig. 1 Essential parts of a flame photometer

i. Fuel gases and their regulation: comprising the fuel reservoir, compressors, pressure regulators and pressure gauges.

ii. Atomizer: consisting, in turn, of the sprayer and the atomisation chamber, where the aerosol is produced and fed into the flame.

iii. Burner: receives the mixture of the combustion gases.

iv. Flame: the true source of emission.

(b) Optical System :

It consists of the optical system for wavelength selection (filters or monochromators), lenses, diaphragms, slits, etc.

(c) Recording System:

It includes detectors like photocells, photo-tubes, photomultipliers, etc., and the electronic means of amplification, measuring and recording.

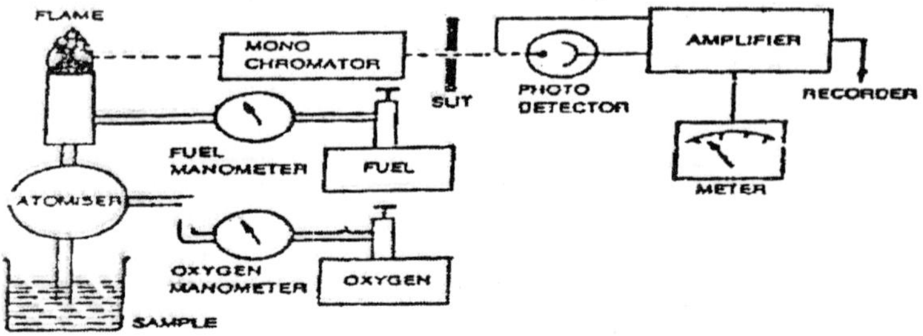

Fig. 2 shows a typical block diagram of a flame photometer.

EMISSION SYSTEM

(a) Fuel Gases and Their Regulation

***Pressure Regulators*:**

In order to obtain a steady emission reading, it is imperative to have a flame that is perfectly steady and free from flickers. To achieve this, the air or oxygen and fuel pressure is maintained constant during the operation of the instrument. Suitable pressure gauges are therefore, provided in the instrument to indicate the pressure actually present in the line. A 25-1b gauge for the oxygen or air supply and a 10-1b gauge for the fuel, are generally used. Pressure regulators are usually followed by needle valves for control of flow. Gauges provided with the regulators are often not sensitive enough to detect small changes of pressure, which have profound effect on the flame photometer operation. Therefore, narrow range pressure regulators and manometers are installed in the line, in order to observe small changes in pressure or gas flow.

Flow Meters:

A flow meter may be inserted in the line from the gas reservoir to the atomizer, in order to detect any clogging of the orifice. For the same flow rate, an appreciable change in the gauge pressure indicates a partially clogged orifice. By controlling the individual flow rates of the fuel and oxygen, the operator can choose various fuel-oxygen mixtures ranging from lean flame mixtures to fuel-

rion types of flames. The flow rates usually vary from 2 to 10 cu. Ft./h.

Fuel Supply:

The fuel gas normally used in flame photometry is the acetylene gas, which is commercially available in cylinders of various sizes. Cylinder acetylene consists of acetylene gas dissolved in acetone, which in turn is adsorbed on a porous filling material. Consequently, after the flame is lit, it should be allowed to burn several minutes before adjustments are attempted in order to vent the excess acetone initially present in the vapour phase. Consumption of acetylene ranges from 1 to 5 cu. Ft./h. The other fuels used in flame photometry are propane, butane and hydrogen. When the available gas pressure is less or is variable, a booster pump is necessary. The pump generally used is a motor driven diaphragm pump, which delivers the gas to the burner at the required volume and pressure.

Oxygen Supply:

Oxygen from cylinders should be supplied to the burner through a regulator capable of delivering approximately 12 cu. Ft./h. at a pressure of 12-15 1b per sq. inch.

Air Supply:

The air supply can be supplied from a cylinder of compressed air or from an air compressor through a tank held at about 10 1b/sq. inch. A pressure compensation valve is placed between the reservoir and the burner. When compressors are used, the air should be filtered through glass wool. Consumption of air is approximately 10 cu. Ft./h. for an acetylene-air flame.

(b) Atomizer:

One of the most exacting problems in the flame photometer design is the manner in which the sample is fed to the flame at an uniform rate. The usual method is to prepare solutions of known concentrations and to spray these into the flame, using some form of aerosol production. Use of an aerosol permits the distribution of the same throughout the body of the flame, rather than its introduction at a single point. In flame photometry, the name atomizer is given to a system which is used to form aerosol by breaking a large mass of liquid into small drops. This little device is responsible for introducing the liquid sample into the flame at a stable and reproducible rate. The atomizer must not be attacked by corrosive solutions.

There are two types of atomizers which are in common use: (i) Those, which introduce the spray into a condensing chamber and into the flame by the air of the combustible gas-air mixture. Large droplets are removed in the condensing chamber. (ii) Those in which the sample is introduced directly into the flame, i.e. the atomizer and the burner are an integral unit.

Figure 3 shows the construction of the first type of atomizer. This is called the discharge-type atomizer and consists of two capillary tubes sealed into the walls of a glass chamber in such a manner that their bores are perpendicular to each other. The sample solution is poured into a funnel on drawn up from a container and is atomized by the blast of air from the tip of the other capillary. However, the atomized stream is composed of coarse spray with large droplets, which condense on the walls of the chamber and helical tube leading to the burner. The condensate flows down to the waste drain. The smaller droplets, in the form of a virtual fog are carried by the air stream into the burner, where it is mixed with the burner gases and carried into the region of active combination. Two removable hypodermic needles of stainless steel or glass are commonly used. With this type of atomizer, the consumption of the sample is comparatively high and ranges between 4 and 25 ml of solution per minute. Of this amount, only 5% actually reaches the flame. The sensitivity of this type of atomizer can be markedly increased by using a chamber which is heated by an electric heater placed around its walls. This hastens the process of vaporisation of the solvent and produces an aerosol of very fine particles, all of which are swept into the burner. In this case, sample consumption is only 0.2 to 0.6 ml min and a substantial portion is carried directly into the burner to yield a much higher sensitivity.

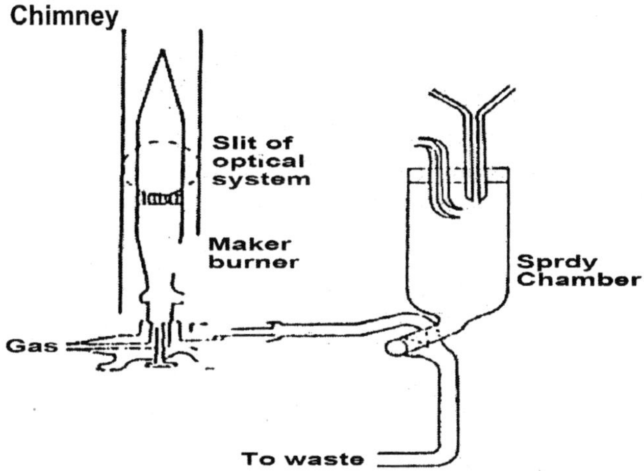

Fig. 3 Discharge type atomizer with condensing chamber and burner

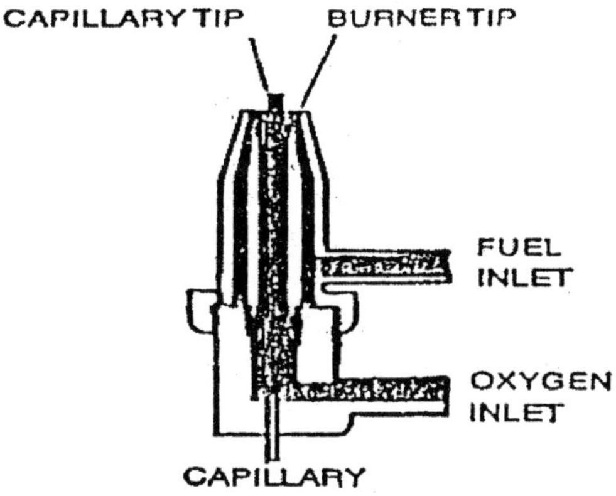

Fig. 4 Integral burner-atomizor

The second type of atomizer is the integral burner atomizer. The unit made of glass or metal is constructed of two concentric tubes. The sample solution is drawn through the innermost tube by the passage of oxygen through the orifice of the middle annulus. At the tip of the inner sample capillary, the liquid is sheared off and dispersed into droplets. The outer annulus supplies the combustible gas to the flame. This type of atomizer is used in Beckman instruments. The body of the unit is machined from brass and the capillary for solution intake is of palladium. All droplets, both large and small, are introduced directly into the flame. Simple consumption is between 0.8 and 2 ml/min. Each atomiser requires separate calibration and is not strictly interchangeable with another of the same type.

Denton and Swartz (1974) maintain that pneumatic nebulisation, though one of the most common methods of aerosol generation, produces a relatively wide droplet size distribution and limited aerosol density. Other techniques, such as the spinning disk aerosol generator, atomizer impactor and isolated droplet generation techniques have also been used, but they produce only very limited concentrations of aerosol. Ultrasonic techniques, when used for aerosol generation, offer unique combination of high solution to aerosol conversion rates, relatively independent of carrier flow gas and have the ability to generate varying sized droplet populations. These workers describe the design of an ultrasonic nebuliser system for the generation of high-density aerosol dispersions.

(c) Burner:

The burner brings the fuel, oxidant and sample aerosol together, so that they may react safely and produce a good flame. Burners used in flame photometry must fulfil the following conditions:

i. When supplied with fuel and oxygen at constant pressure, the shape, size and temperature of the flame will remain constant.

ii. Assist in a perfect distribution of the mixture of gases and the aerosol, which carries the atomized solution under analysis.

iii. Have a tip of suitable shape to produce a symmetrical flame and ensure a homogeneous flow and distribution of the gases, avoiding a strike-back in the burner from accidental fluctuations in the feed system.

iv. Prevent condensation of the aerosol in the stem of the burner, which would reduce the effective quantity of the sample brought into the flame.

The most commonly used burner for low temperature flames is Meker type. Here, the fuel-gas issues from a small orifice and passes through a venturi throat, where considerable air is entrained. The mixture of gas and the entrained air passes up the burner tube and burns at the top of the burner, where the combustion is assisted by the surrounding air.

A deep grid of metal across the mouth of the burner prevents the flame from striking back down the tube. To screen the flame from air drafts, it is surrounded by a glass chimney, which also protects the operator.

In the integral burner-atomizer unit, the sample solution is introduced directly into the flame. A cut section of this type of burner is shown in Fig. 4.

(d) Flame:

The flame is the most important part of the flame photometer, since it forms the source in which the light radiations characteristic of the elements under analysis are produced. The flame performs the following functions:

i. It converts the constituents of the sample to be analysed from the liquid or solid state into gaseous state

ii. Decomposes these constituents into atoms or simpler molecules.

iii. Excites the resulting atomic or molecular species to emit light radiations.

In order to produce accurate results, the flame must be very stable. If its temperature or structure shows a change over a period of time, the emission produced by a given sample will also change.

The flame temperature must be high enough to excite the atoms to higher energy levels, so that emission may take place. In general, the flames are produced by burning the gases given in Table 1:

Table 1 Flame Temperature °C

Fuel	*In Air*	*In Oxygen*
Propane	1925	2800
Butane	1900	2900
Hydrogen	2100	2780
Acetylene	2200	3050

All the fuels employed in flame emission spectroscopy produce both continuous background as well as certain band spectra. The nature and intensity of the spectrum for a given fuel is strongly dependent upon fuel-to-oxidant ratio and the flame temperature.

OPTICAL SYSTEM:

The complex light emission produced in the flame by a solution containing one or more elements, makes it necessary to select the radiations of different wavelengths for each of the elements present in the solution. This job is accomplished by the optical system, which collects the light from the steadiest part of the flame, renders it monochromatic and then focuses it on to the surface of the photodetector. A concave mirror is often placed behind the flame, with its centre of curvature in the flame. In this way, the intensity of the emitted light is nearly doubled.

Filters:

Wavelength selection may be done by optical filters or monochromators. Less expensive instruments make use of filters, which may be absorption type or interference type. The usual glass or gelatin absorption filters have wide spectral bandwidths – 35 to 45 mμ in width at one-half the maximum transmittance. Their overall transmittance is only 5-25%, decreasing with improved spectral isolation. Absorption filters do not give the degree of monochromaticity required for analysing complex systems and hence, the flame photometers so equipped are restricted in use to the determination of only sodium, potassium, calcium and lithium.

To improve the resolution, interference filters are often used. They are the most suitable for flame photometry as compared with absorption filters, because they allow a much narrower band of wavelengths to pass. They are similar to monochromators in selectivity, but are less expensive. Standard interference filters having spectral bandwidths from 10 to 17 mμ at one-half the maximum transmittance are commercially available. The same characteristics are shown by continuous wedge filters, which allow a continuous selection of different wavelengths. The continuity of an interference filter is achieved by using a spacer film of graded thickness between the two semi-transparent layers of silver. These filters usually have a working interval of 400 to 700 nm. They provide a dispersion of 5.5 nm/mm, with a transmittance which is usually not higher than 35%.

Monochromators:

Monochromators are incorporated in the instruments, which are expected to provide better isolation of spectral energy. This requirement emanates when the spectrum lines are very close or very weak or both. By using narrow slit widths and sensitive detecting circuits, quite narrow bands of radian energy can be isolated. There are two means of dispersing radiation – by refraction or by interference. The examples of the two types are prism monochromator and diffraction grating, respectively. In flame photometry, prism monochromators have been most widely accepted. They may be of glass or quartz. The glass prisms are only suitable for emissions essentially in the visible region, whereas the quartz prisms enable many atomic lines to be studied, that occur in the far ultraviolet region of the spectrum. In prism monochromators, emission bands or lines are chosen by local selection with movable exit slits or by prism rotation, where all the lines of the spectrum are passed through a fixed slit one after the other. The wavelength scale is non-linear as in prism spectrographs.

Dispersal of light may also be obtained by means of diffraction in a grating. A grating is produced by ruling grooves at extremely close intervals, of the order of 15,000 grooves per inch, on a highly polished surface. The dispersion is linear, which permits a constant bandwidth to be used throughout the spectrum. The wavelength scale in this case is linear.

For the analysis of complex spectra, the resolving power should be very high. Resolving power is a measure of the ability of the monochromator to resolve two closely spaced lines of about equal intensity. Perhaps, the most straight test of an instrument's resolving power concerns the separation of the manganese line at 403.3 nm, the potassium line at 404.4 nm and the lead line at 405.8 nm from each other.

RECORDING SYSTEM:

Photosensitive Detectors:

After the isolation of the lines or bands emitted by the chemical elements under analysis in the optical system, the light intensities of these radiations have to be measured quantitatively. This is done by causing the radiation selected to fall on a photosensitive element. The electric current produced is then measured with a galvanometer, either directly or after amplification. The intensity of electric current produced is a function of the concentration of the solution under analysis. The photodetectors are either of photovoltaic or photoemissive type.

Photovoltaic cells have very little internal resistance and the current they produce cannot be amplified by dc amplifiers. The current is measured directly by connecting the terminals of the cell to a highly sensitive galvanometer. The spectral response of a selenium cell adequately covers various wavelengths encountered in the analysis of common alkali and alkaline earth metals. The sensitivity that can be achieved with these cells is considerable, as they give currents of more than 5×10^{-10} A, when they receive a light flux of more than 10^{-6} lumen.

Selenium cells are highly sensitive to temperature variations. The cells have a certain inertia and at least a quarter of an hour must be allowed for them to settle, with the burner lit before the readings are taken. A fall in efficiency, due to aging is a well known characteristic of these cells and they are also subject to fatigue upon exposure to prolonged illumination.

Phototubes of several types may also be used for detecting the radiations. They differ essentially from barrier layer cells, in that they need and external electrical supply to provide a sufficient potential between the electrodes. Phototubes are less sensitive than barrier layer cells and the current produced usually needs amplification. Since they exhibit large internal resistance, amplification of the cathode current by an external circuit can be conveniently done.

The preferred detector for weak light intensities is the photomultiplier tube. This is many times more sensitive than the simple phototube, which in turn, permits greater spectral resolution without loss of signals. They are available with envelopes of ordinary glass or with quartz window inserts for use in the ultraviolet region below 350 nm.

Electrical Circuits:

The final step in recording the light radiations produced in the source of emission consists in transforming the electrical signal produced by the selected radiation in the photosensitive element into a reading, by which is related to the concentration of the solution under analysis.

Single-Beam Instruments:

For selenium photocells, a spotlight, multi-reflection galvanometer is quite suitable. The galvanometer may possess a maximum sensitivity ranging from 0.007 to 0.0004 μA \ mm scale division and a coil resistance of approximately 400 Ω. As the cells are generally of low resistance when illuminated, rather low values of resistance must be external circuit. Figure 5 shows a simple arrangement for measuring directly the output of a single barrier-layer cell. This type of circuit is suitable for a single-beam instrument, which contains only one set of optics. The photoelectric current generated in the photocell by the light is given to the galvanometer through the coarse and fine sensitivity controls at B and A respectively. Selenium cells exhibit no dark current, which would require suppression, but a suppressor circuit might be useful in bucking out a reading resulting from the flame background.

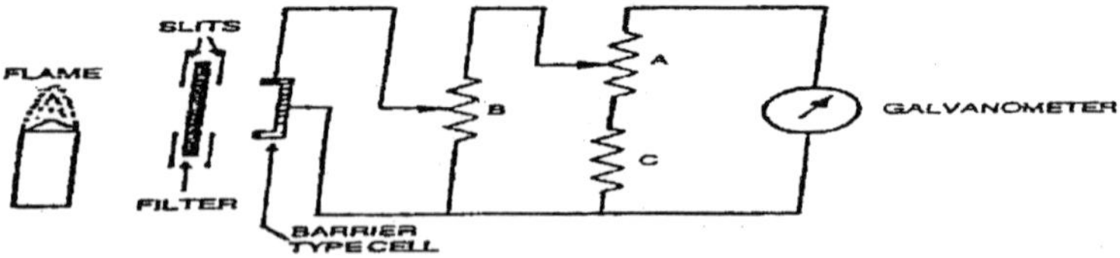

Fig. 5 Circuit diagram for single-beam direct-reading flame photometer

Double-Beam Instruments

In double-beam instruments, provision is made for a second light path, which is emitted by an internal standard element. The internal standard and unknown wavelengths are isolated by means of optical filters in a dual optical system, and each beam is focused on a photoelectric cell (Fig. 6). The circuit is so arranged that the photoelectric currents produced by the emitted radiations of the unknown and internal standard elements oppose each other through a galvanometer. By means of an accurate potentiometer (P_1), the opposing photoelectric currents can be balanced. The settings of the potentiometer required to produce balance, are calibrated in terms of known solutions. Sensitivity adjustments are made with another potentiometer (P_2) by shunting currents generated by the measuring cell. This makes it possible to read more concentrated solutions of the test element without changing the concentration of the internal standard used.

Circuits used with Photomultiptier Tubes:

The output current from the last amplifying stage in a photomultiplier tube for many solutions and concentration ranges normally employed, often lie between 10 and 100 μA and can be directly measured by a spotlight galvanometer (Fig. 7), or simply a rugged pointer type micrometer. Photomultiplier tubes possess an appreciable output current even when the tube is dark, and therefore, for direct measurements it will be necessary to carry out a background correction before measurement. This is done by compensating with an auxiliary battery and adjusting R_2. The sensitivity of the photomultiplier tube can be adjusted by varying the voltage per dynode or preferably by variation of the voltage applied to the first dynode.

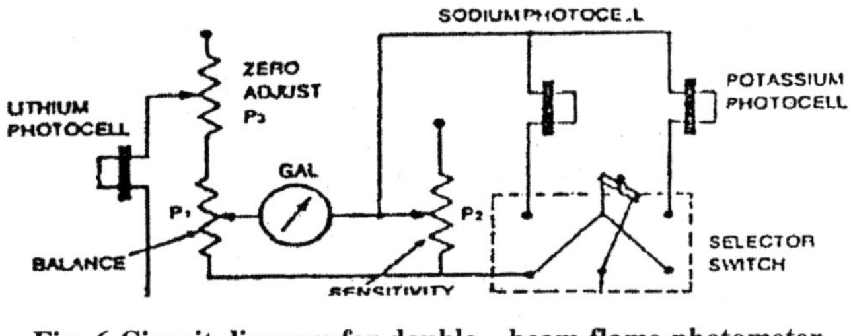

Fig. 6 Circuit diagram for double—beam flame photometer

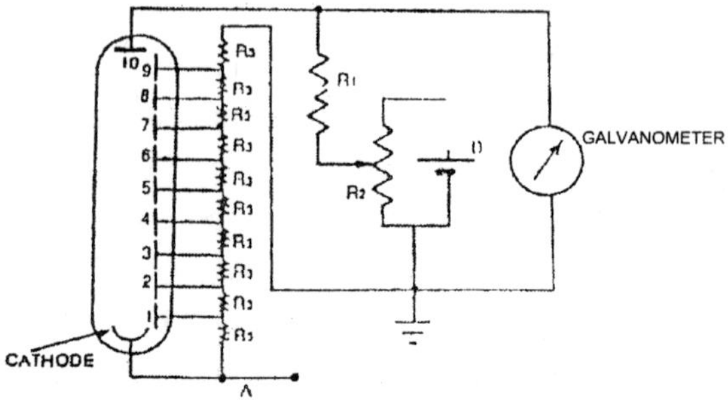

Fig. 7 Circuit for direct reading flame photometer using a photomultiplier tube

Amplifier for phototube Circuits:

The current form the phototube is generally so small that it is necessary to amplify it, quite often by of 10^5 to 10^6. The amplification of a direct current can be achieved with the help of vacuum tube amplifiers, with special electrometer tubes, or other vacuum tubes operating under electrometer conditions used in first stage. Vacuum tube amplifiers are voltage operated devices and therefore the changes of phototube current must be converted to voltage changes by having a resistance series with the phototube. This resistance is usually kept very high and is of the order of 10,000 MΩ. The amplifiers are throughout direct coupled. A serious drawback of dc amplifiers is the zero drift, which is a slow, continuous shift of the galvanometer pointer. DC amplifiers are also sensitive to various in supply voltage and temperature changes. Although amplifier circuits consisting of vacuum tubes are still found in the instruments, integrated circuits with high input impedance are now available, which have greatly simplified the circuit construction.

Amplifiers for Photomultiplier Tube Circuits:

Though the photomultiplier tube itself provides a large amplification, this can be appreciably increased by an amplifying circuit. The last dynode of the photomultiplier tube is usually connected to the grid of the amplifying valve and at the same time to a grid leak, thus causing a potential difference, the variations of which are amplified.

In order to reduce the rapid and random fluctuations, a long enough time constant is incorporated in the amplifier circuit to aid in the integrating process, and thus the meter is rendered unresponsive to sudden flashes of light in the flame. Usually, the time constant is chosen to be approximately 1 s and is obtained by connecting a capacitor in parallel with the coupling resistor. To overcome the problem of drift of dc amplifiers, the light from the flame can be interrupted, and the photoelectric current can be amplified by an ac amplifier. A synchronously rotating disc is placed before the flame and the photoelectric current is thus converted to a chopped dc signal, which can then be amplified by an ac amplifier.

Figure 8 shows a circuit diagram using solid state components, which can be used to amplify current obtained in a photomultiplier. The output of the PMT is applied to the gate of FET Q_1. Q_1 inverts this negative going signal to positive and applies this to the non-inverting side of operational amplifier Z_1. Due to divider network R_9 and R_8, the gain of the operational amplifier Z_1 is held at 10. The output of the circuit can be directly connected to a moving coil meter.

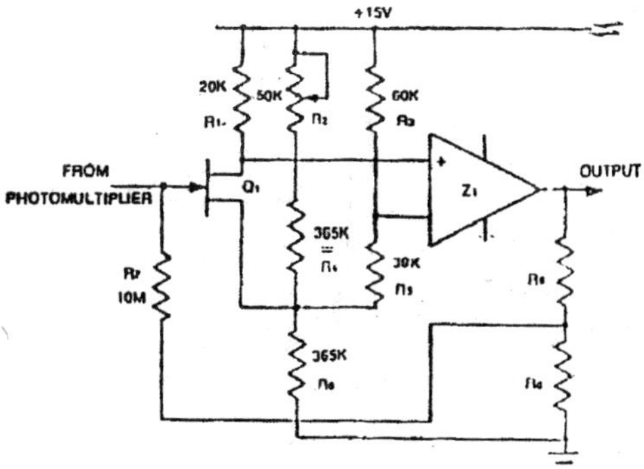

Fig. 8 Typical amplifier circuit used in flame photometer

Digital display type flame photometers are now available in which the analog voltage is converted to digital form and then given to Nixic tubes or LEDs for numerical display.

CLINICAL FLAME PHOTOMETERS:

The flame photometer is one of the most useful instruments in clinical analyses. This is due to the suitability of the flame photometer for determining sodium, potassium and calcium, which are of immense importance in the development of the living being and indispensable to its physiological functions. In the clinical analysis of sodium and potassium, the flame photometer gives, rapidly and accurately, numerous differential data for normal and pathological values.

KLiNa Flame System of M/s. Beckman is a dedicated instrument for simultaneous analysis of sodium and potassium. In this instrument, sample handling is automatic, as the system has a turntable, which will hold up to 20 samples in cups and an automatic positive piston displacement dilutor, that dilutes the sample prior to entering the spray chamber (Figs. 9 & 10).

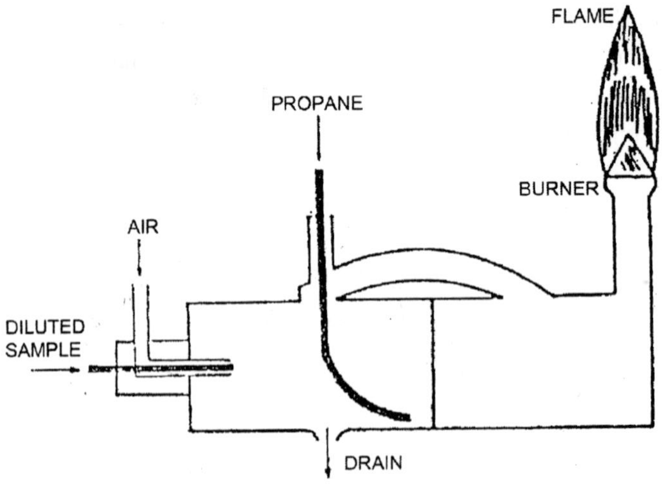

Fig. 9 Flame spray chambers and burner of KLiNa flame photometer

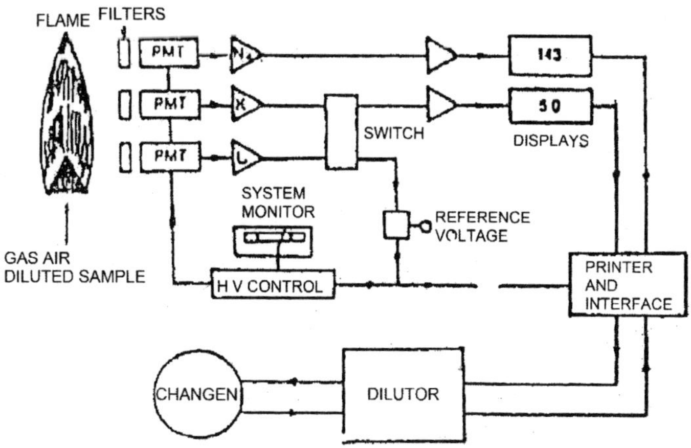

Fig. 10 Schematic diagram of Beckman KLiNa flame photometer

Commercial Designs:

Figure 11 shows the general arrangement of the EEL flame photometer. Air is introduced round the atomiser nozzle through the inlet (F) at a controllable pressure. The pressure is indicated by a pressure gauge provided on the front panel of the instrument. Gas enters the mixing chamber through the tube (M) and is likewise controllable. The air flow round the atomiser is applied to draw the sample (B) up the capillary tube (C) and through the atomiser, which injects it in a fine spray into the mixing chamber (D). Larger droplets failing from the air-stream pass through the drain tube (E). The baffles (G) produce an even mixture of gas, air and sample, which passes to the burner (L) and is ignited, to burn with a broad, flat flame within a well-ventilated chimney.

INTERFERENCES IN FLAME PHOTOMETRY:

Flame photometry is subject to several types of interferences, which arise during the course of analysis through variations in any of the parts of the instrumental system, or in the composition of the samples. These interferences give rise to experimental errors. Some of these interferences are:

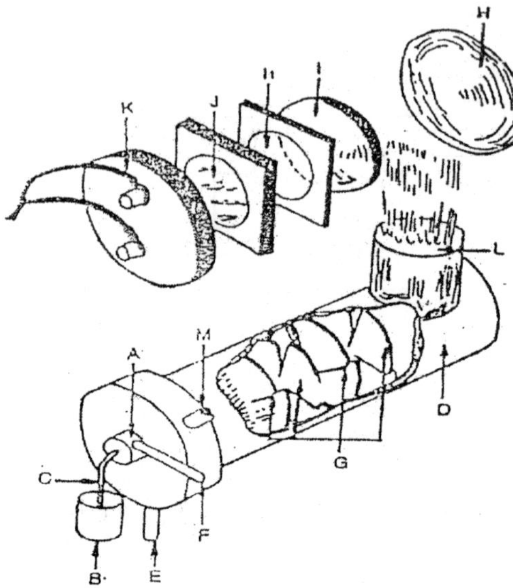

Fig.11 General arrangement of the atomizer, combustion Chamber and optical system of EEL flame photometer

Flame Background Emission:

A flame is an extremely complex mixture of reacting gases. Since these gases are hot, they emit a certain amount of light, even when no sample atoms have been injected into the flame. This light is the flame background. The lines produced by a sample are superimposed on this background. Failure to correct properly for the background reading can be a source of serious error. It is desirable to eliminate, as far as possible, flame background and other emission lines from the measurements. The narrower the bandwidth of the monochromator used, the more efficient is this elimination.

Direct Spectral Interference:

This interference occurs when the emission lines are so close together that the monochromator cannot separate them. For example, the emission of the orange band of CAOH interferes with the sodium line at 589 nm. Interference is more serious when absorption filters are used in place of monochromators. In this case, the two lines overlap partially or completely, and will be read together in proportion to the degree of overlap. If the interference cannot be obviated by increased resolution, the difficulty must be overcome by prior removal of one element, perhaps by selective solvent extraction.

Self-Absorption:

Interference due to self-absorption occurs due to the absorption of radiant energy through collision with atoms of its own kind present in the ground energy level. If some of the radiant energy is self-absorbed, the strength of the spectral line is weakened. Self-absorption primarily depends upon the number of atoms present in the ground state, the concentration of atomised solution and by the probability that these atoms will be excited by the incident radiation from excited atoms of its own kind. Self-absorption is insignificant at very low concentrations of a test element.

Effect of Anions:

Anionic disturbances result from a radiation in the number of free metallic ions by stable combination in the flame with the anions. There is usually no interference with concentrations less than 0.1 M. Above this concentration, sulphuric, nitric and phosphoric acids, in particular, show a marked effect in lowering metallic emission. For example, the strong depression of the calcium emission in the presence of phosphate, aluminate and other similar anions has been fairly well known. In practice, over limited intervals of concentration, the depression is linear and this forms the basis for indirect determination of the depressant in the presence of a standard amount of calcium.

Effect of Ionisation:

The easily excitable alkali metals, such as potassium show the phenomenon of ionisation through excessive dissociation and consequently result in the depletion of the number of available neutral atoms that can be excited. This in turn, weakens the intensity of the atomic spectrum, whereas any ionic spectrum is strengthened. When small quantities of easily ionised metals are added to a flame, the number of neutral atoms tends to increase more rapidly in comparison to the ionised atoms, in proportion to the concentration of metal sprayed into the flame. As a result, the curve of intensity versus concentration may initially be concave upward.

Solution Characteristics:

The physical properties of the solutions strongly influence the atomisation rate, which in turn influences the luminescence of the flame. The main factors responsible for this are the differences in viscosity, surface tension, density, volatility and temperature between standards and samples. For example, an increase in viscosity lowers the atomisation rate, with a consequent weakening of the emission, causing errors and loss of sensitivity. Similarly, variation in surface tension is considered as another source of error. They affect the emission in a similar manner to viscosity, through their effect on atomising conditions. Added salts and acids hinder the evaporation of solvent, large droplets result in a diminished quantity of aerosol reaching the burner, because the larger droplets are more likely to settle upon the walls of the condensing chamber.

There are several standard ways of eliminating or avoiding the influence of the above mentioned factors. The techniques of overcoming interferences demand high skill and experience. With the development of atomic absorption spectrophotometry, in which the problems of interference and flame stability are not as severe, flame emission analysis has been largely limited to the determination of sodium, potassium and less frequently lithium, calcium, manganese and copper in relatively simple mixtures.

PROCEDURE FOR DETERMINATIONS:

Calibration Curve Method:

In order to determine the concentration of an unknown element X in a given sample, or a series of samples, the instrument is first standardised by making a calibration curve. For this, it is desirable to know the probable range of concentration of X in the sample, so that a series of calibration standards can be made up; having a suitable spread over the range expected. The instrument is first adjusted to give a zero meter reading, when pure distilled water is aspirated into the flame. The instrument settings are then adjusted to give the full-scale reading, with the most concentrated standard sample. Without altering this adjustment, emission intensifies for the remaining standards and the unknown are measured. Calibration curves are thus plotted and the concentrations read off against this calibration.

A background correction to the calibration data can be made with a spectrophotometer by measuring the radiation intensity on either side of the peak at points sufficiently removed, so that the line spectrum contributes nothing to the radiation. Otherwise, the background is estimated from a blank containing all components of the sample, except the one being determined. Instrument response is proportional to the concentration, and hence a straight line is obtained. The concentration of the unknown is obtained from the calibrated curve.

Since it is difficult to obtain a flame of high long-term stability, it is usual to check the calibration at frequent intervals by spraying a standard. This ensures that drift can be measured and taken into account. In fact calibration curves are difficult to reproduce on the same day; virtually impossible on different days.

The concentrations to which the samples are diluted for measurement can often be selected, if the concentration in the original solution is much greater than the detection limit of the element concerned. Careful choice of the concentration is very important, as it has a considerable effect on the accuracy for analysis for the following reasons:

i) Calibration curves are not necessarily linear. It is found that the curves for a given element are linear over a limited range. At stronger concentrations, the same element would give a curved calibration.

ii) In case of a high total concentration of solids in the flame, the flame background is greatly increased and the burner may be fouled.

iii) If the viscosity of the sample is too high, it may not spray efficiently.

iv) If the solution is diluted excessively, errors of dilution may occur and the signal-to-noise ratio may decrease.

Standard Addition Method:

A number of radiation interferences can be avoided by using the method of standard addition. In this method, net emission readings are obtained on two solutions, solution A containing an aliquot of the unknown solution and solution B containing the same quantity of unknown solution plus a measured amount of a standard solution of the element. The amount of test element in each of the two solutions is then determined from their measured emission intensifies and the standard calibration curve. Subtracting the quantity of unknown found in solution A from that found in solution B, gives the amount of test element equal to that added; when there is no depression or enhancement. When one of these effects is present, the corrections are applied, which correct for the interference. It is necessary that the calibration curve be linear over the range of concentrations employed.

Internal Standard Method:

The flame system is a critical part of the Flame photometer and its long-term stability is dependant upon :(i) fuel flow, (ii) air pressure,

(iii) nebulisation rate, (iv) burner / atomising chamber temperature. While the first two factors can be controlled effectively to within acceptable limits by suitable instrument design, the other two are placed easily controlled in this way. To overcome variation from these sources, internal standard procedure has been developed.

In these methods a fixed quantity of the internal standard element is added to the blank sample and standard solution. The radiation of the element is measured together with those of the elements under analysis by dual detectors, or be scanning successively the two emission lines. The ratio of the emission intensity of the analysis lying to that of the internal standard line is plotted against the concentration of the analysis of the element on log-log paper, to prepare the calibration curve for the number of standards. Corrections for background radiations are made for each line. The plot of log (emission ratio) verses log (concentration of test element) will produced a straight line, whose. slope ideally is 45^0 over limited concentration intervals. On most double beam instruments, this ratio is given by the reading of the balancing potentiometer. Calibration curves may be drawn on a linear co-ordinate paper. A ratio, rather than an absolute light intensity that is being measured, because of which fluctuations due to variable operation of the nebuliser-burner systems; are greatly minimised. This procedure also reduces errors due to differences in the composition of the test and standard solutions. ,

The choice of a suitable element and spectral line depends upon the following analytical conditions

(i) The element should give spectral lines that are closed to those of the analysis element, so that it is not necessary to use a different type of photo detector. Thus, lithium 671 nM line is a suitable reference for the analysis of potassium at 761 nM and sodium at 589 nM, but it is less satisfactory for the determination of calcium at 422.7 nM.

ii) The element must be one that is not present in the samples and must available in a high state of purity.

iii) It must be added in concentrations very near to those of the analysis element, so that radiation of approximately equal intensifies may be obtained. For this reason, the concentration of lithium is normally adjusted to 100 mg/ cm^3 (15 mEq), in solutions where the sodium and potassium concentration fie in the 0 to 100 μg/cm^3 rage.

iv) The reference element must produce radiations that are perfectly selectable.

v) When added, the element must not alter the physical properties of the solution.

For analysis of alkali metals and even of other elements, lithium has been preferred as an internal standard, as it satisfies most of the above mentioned requirements.

MAINTENANCE FLAME PHOTOMETER:

Routine, regular maintenance and functional checks are essential for any type of flamephotometer.

1. Nebuilizer (Atomiser) should be periodically cleaned with cleaning wire for clogs and any other obstructions.
2. Flow rate pf nebuilizer should be optimised in such a way that spray should be fine without any droplets and it should be consume 2-3 mi/min.
3. Burner head and capillary should be flushed with water daily to remove salt deposits.
4. The burner assembly, chimney and optical modules like filter, lenses should be checked for dirt and film accumulated and cleaned at periodic intervals.

10

NEPHALOMETER AND TURBIDIMETER

INTRODUCTION TO TURBIDITY MEASUREMENTS:

Turbidity is defined as the expression of optical property that causes light to be scattered and absorbed rather than transmitted in straight lenes through the sample. This scatting and absorption is caused by the interaction of light with particles suspended in the sample media. Turbidity can be caused by suspended solids including silt, clay, algae and other plankton, microbes, organic matter and other fine, insoluble particles. Particles interfering with light transmittance cause the sample to take on a hazy or cloudy appearance. Simply put, turbidity is the opposite of clarity.

The methods of measurement of turbidity fall under tree classes:

(i) Measurement of the ratio of intensities of scattered and incident light.

(ii) Measurement of the ratio of intensities of transmitted and incident light.

(iii) Measurement of extinction effect i.e. the depth at which a target disappears beneath the layer of a turbid medium.

Turbidity originally was determined by measuring the depth of a column of liquid required to cause the image of a candle flame at the bottom to diffuse into a uniform glow. This was known as the Jackson candle turbidimeter. Calibration was based on suspensions o silica from Fuller's or diatomaceous earth. The turbidity caused by 1 ppm of suspended silica was defined as one Jackson Turbidity Unit (JTU).

Turbidity usually is measured today by applying nephelometry, a technique to measure the level of light scattered by particles at right angles to the incident light beam. When the light is incident on a particle, the energy is scattered in all directions. The scattered in all directions. The scattered level is proportional to the particulate concentration and can be measured readily by an electronic photometer. Photodetectors are available with a very high sensitivity to allow measurement of low turbidities.

Turbidity of a liquid is important for many reasons, depending on its use. Besides aesthetic appeal of crystal-clear water, low turbidity is important in drinking water to minimize water-borne pathogens. Turbidity in water can be caused by harmful organisms, particles that feed them or particles that can shelter them from disinfection processes. To assure a safe drinking water supply, water plants are required by law to maintain a uniform low turbidity in their finished product.

In other liquids, turbidity can be caused by particulates detrimental to the end use, or perhaps by particles that are a vital ingredient of a product. In either case, turbidity can be used as a quality control measure to monitor the efficiency of the treatment of manufacturing process.

LABORATORY TURBIDITMETER:

Laboratory turbidimeter, manufactured by several firms, like M/s HACH model 2100A, operate on the basis of nephelometry, and measure the amount of light scattered from a directed beam by particulates in the sample (Fig. 1). Light from the source is directed up through the bottom of a special flat-bottom cell containing the sample. As light beam strikes particles in the sample, some of the light is scattered at right angles to the light path and is received by the detector, e.g. a photomultiplier tube. The PMT converts the light energy to an electrical signal which is indicated on the meter. PMTs are very sensitive to UV light scattered by minute particles (0.1 to 0.5 microns), making the instrument suitable for, for instance, monitoring highly filtered water.

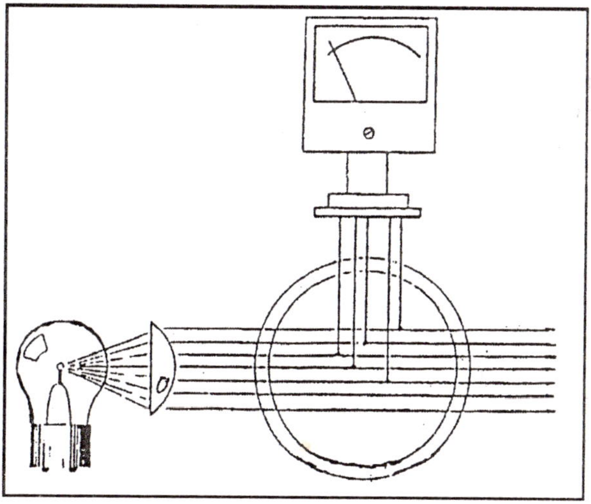

Fig.1 Nephelometric turbidimeter and its specifications

CALIBRATION AND STANDARDIZATION:

For convenient routine calibration of the turbidimeter, secondary standards in different ranges between 0 and 1000 Nephelometric Turbidity Units (NTU). Calibration against a primary reference standard is based on a polymer suspension of formazin (FTU).

MAINTENANCE :

Maintenance requirements for turbiditimeters are minimal. Lamp can be replaced easily after their useful life is over. Cleaning sample cells thoroughly after every use, and periodic calibration are the only other requirements. Usually, the solid-state electronics is designed for high reliability and all components are operated below their rated voltages for extended life.

PORTABLE INSTRUMENTS :

These instruments resemble the laboratory instruments in their principle of operation and construction. The amount of scattered light is directly proportional to the sample's turbidity. These instruments are for on-site turbidity testing with the accuracy of laboratory meters. They are powered by rechargeable nickel cadmium batteries. A rugged plastic case provides space for sample cells, calibration standards, and battery charger. Overnight charging the battery pack provides approximately 10 hours of continuous operation. Calibration is carried out in the same way as that for laboratory instruments.

RATIO TURBIDIMETER:

A ratio turbidimeter is a more sophisticated variation of a normal nephlometric turbidimeter. Its light path diagram is shown in Fig. 2. Its unique optical system can measure turbidity caused by suspended particulates in virtually and fluid, regardless of sample colour. A suitable detector system design is incorporated to minimize stray light. Industrial producers can obtain reliable quality control data on the clarity of coloured liquids such as beverages, chemicals, cosmetics, pharmaceuticals, cleaning solutions, petroleum products, etc. as well as water.

Light is focused into a narrow beam before being passed through the sample contained in a glass cell. In particle-free samples, the light is transmitted through the sample to the transmitted light detector. The transmitted light level represents the total amount of light available for turbidity measurements and provides automatic compensation for light energy absorbed by a coloured sample.

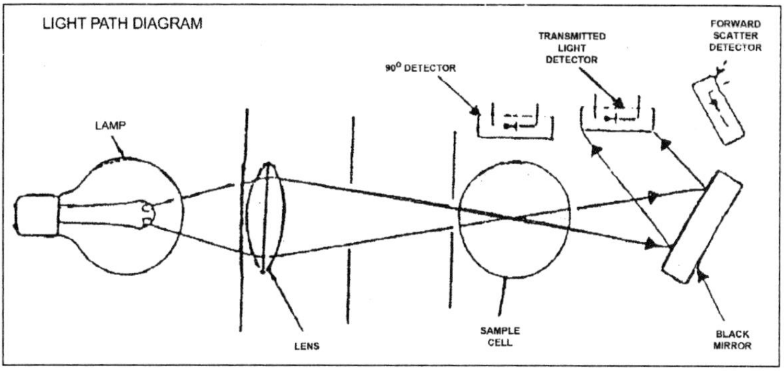

Fig. 2 Optical diagram of a ratio turbidimeter

Light scattered by particles in the sample, is received by the 90° - scatter detector. This signal is proportional to the level of particulates in the sample. As particle levels increase, light is also scattered at acute angles to the light beam. This is called forward scattered light as it continues in generally the same direction as the incident beam. This is received by the forward scatter detector and factored against the transmitted light signal to provide a linear response to turbidity over a wide range of sample turbidity.

The output of the detector system is a ratio of the 90° - scatter detector to an electronically weighted sum of the transmitted and forward scatter detector signals. This ratio optical system also provides excellent reading stability and automatically compensates for lamp fluctuations, haze and dust on the optics, and temperature coefficients of detectors and amplifiers, A 0-1 volt output can be included to drive standard chart recorder for permanent records and trend indication. A flow- through cell assembly for monitoring continuous flow and recirculating sample streams is also available from some manufactures (e.g. HACH model 18900 -10).

Digital display eliminates reading errors and reads to nearest 0.01 NTU on the 0-2 NTU range. Calibration drift is minimized. Due to its stability, there is little need for day-to-day standardization. Weekly check with secondary turbidity standards are sufficient to maintain calibration accuracy.

SURFACE SCATTER TURBIDITMETER:

The forward scatter turbidimeter is especially useful for on-line measurement of turbidity as it eliminates many of the problems associated with conventional on-line instruments. This stems from the absence of contact between the sample and optical system components. It is suitable for a wide variety of water and wastewater treatment processes. The salient features of the surface scatter turbiditmeter are:

- There is no contact between the liquid and optical components. Virtually no cleaning is required.
- Both very high and very low turbidities can be measured.
- Wetted parts are made of corrosion-resistant materials for extended life. Electronics is isolated in a sealed compartment.
- A reflectance plate serves as a secondary standard providing a fixed reference for routine standardization.
- Two independently adjustable alarm relays and analog outputs can be used to record turbidity levels and initiate action of external control and/ or annunciator devices.
- A wide selection of recorder output is provided. A current output card can be installed to provide a selection of 0-20 mA, 4-20 mA or 10-50 mA in place of the voltage output.

PRINCIPLE OF OPERATION:

The flow diagram given in Fig. 3 illustrates the surface scatter method of turbidity measurement. Sample is brought into the centre of a diagonal turbidimeter body. Rising to the top, the sample overflows a weir into a drain ring forming an optically flat surface. A light beam is focused on the liquid surface art an acute angle. Suspended particles in the sample will scatter light in proportion to the sample turbidity. A silicon photodiode detector mounted directly above the liquid surface detects the level of scattered light, converting it to an electric signal which is displayed on the instrument meter. The angled turbidimeter body serves to trap refracted light and collect settleable solids where they can be purged through the bottom drain.

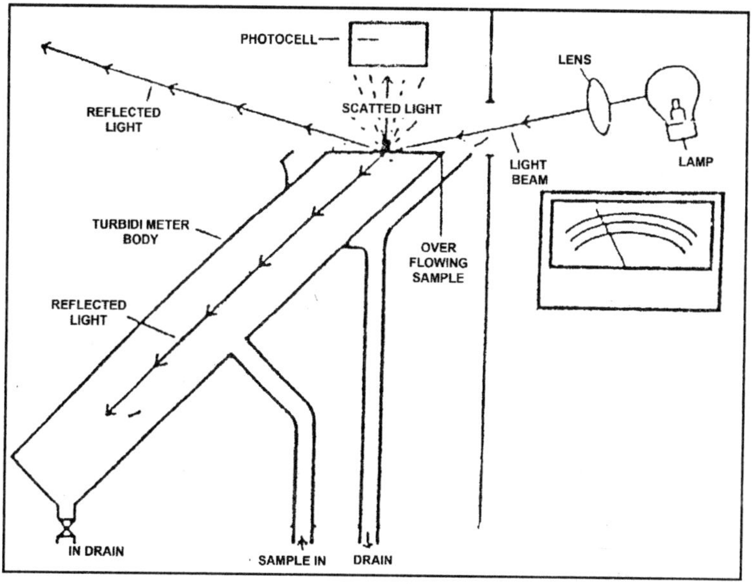

Fig. 3 Schematic flow diagram of a forward scatter turbidimeter

CALIBRATION AND STANDARDIZATION:

The meter is calibrated in NTU for five separate measuring ranges: 0-1.0, 0.10, 1-100, 1-1000, and 0-5000 NTU. Calibration is based on the primary standard formazin. The reflectance plate secondary standard can be used to detect and compensate for changes in standardization. Typical specifications of a forward scatter turbiditmeter are given below.

Specification:

Ranges	0-1.0 NTU, 0.10:0, 0.100, 0-1,000, 0-5,000
Accuracy/ Reproducibility	± 5% of full scale ± 2 % of full scale
Resolution	0.05 NTU on 0-1.0 range
Stray Light	Less than 0.04 NTU
Sample requ ired	1 to 2 liters/ min (15-20 gph)
Sample Pressure	1 psig to maintain flow rate requirements
Resource Time	30 sec to detect change
Recorder Outputs	Selectable voltage output of 0-10mV, 0-100mV, 0-1mV and 0-10mV. Minimum impedance of 50K ohms. Current output of 0-20 mA, 4-20 mA or 1 0-50 mA are selectable with output card provided
Alarm	Dual set points fully adjustable over the operating range. SPDT contacts rated for 3A at 115 Vac, resistive load. Red LED local panel indicators show alaram status.
Light Source	Tungsten, lamp, estimated life 7,000 hrs
Sensor	Silicon photodiode
Operating Temperature Range	1-50°C (33-122°F)
Power requirements	115/230 Vac, 50/60 Hz, 60 W switch convertible
Construction	Epoxy-coated steel enclosure meets NEMA -12 type dust and splash-proof requirements wetted parts of PVC and latex

TURBIDITY STANDARDS:

One of the earliest calibration scale for turbidity measurements was based on suspension of weighed amounts of silica in distilled water. 1 TU was established as the turbidity resulting from a suspension of 1 ppm of silica. These standards are difficult to reproduce a reasonable degree of accuracy.

Today, the accepted primary standard for turbidity is a preparation of formazin as its synthesis can be reproduced from pure chemical compounds. Formazin is prepared by making a solution of 5.00 g of primary standard grade hydrazine sulphate (N_2H_4 + H_2 SO_4) and 50.0 g of hexamethylenetetramine [$(CH_2)_6$ N_4] and dilution to 1 liter with pure water. Standing at room temperature (25°C) for 24 hours, the solution will develop a white particulate suspension. This suspension is defined as 4000 turbidity units, FTU.

This solution can be reproduced with high accuracy. Working standards of desired turbidity are prepared from dilutions of the 4000 TU stock. The 4000-TU formazin suspensions are stable for long periods of time while dilutions used as working standards are not. It is recommended that dilute working standards should be prepared freshly from the 4000-TU stock.

PREPARATION OF FORMAZIN:

Fromazin is an aqueous suspension of an insoluble polymer formed by the condensation reaction between hydrazine sulfate and hexanethylenetetramine:

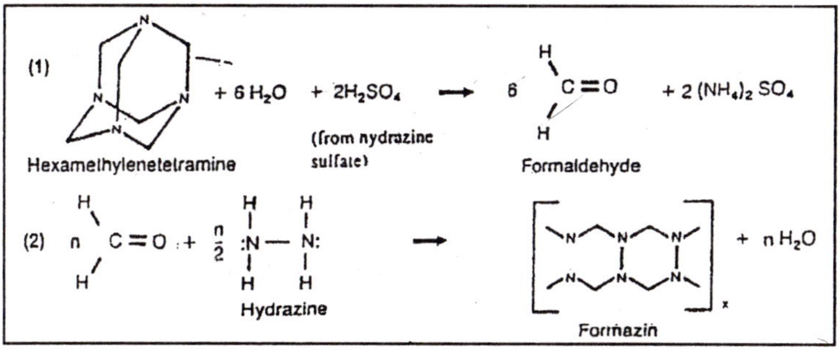

TURBIDIMETERY: USES

- Maintaining uniformity of peppermint oil used as a flavoring.

- Monitoring precipitates in chilling brine water.
- Monitoring resins and paints for foreign particles that may result in premature failure of the coating.
- Detecting barium nitrate particles in rust inhibitors.
- Monitoring silver nitrate solution to control silver content.
- Detecting changes in cell sizes of body cell tissue (a medical research application)
- Monitoring filter efficiency in manufacturing stainless steel filters.
- Detecting the presence and changing sizes of carbon particles in clear liquids
- Monitoring red water problems in community water distribution systems (A portable turbidimeter application).
- Assuring the proper proportion of ingredients as a quality control measure in the manufacture of synthetic fibers.
- Detecting undisolved additives in motor oil through turbidity measurements (More rapid then a sedimentation test).
- Detecting trace contaminants in high fructose syrup.
- Monitoring the clarity of mild acids (paper mill application).
- Monitoring the filtrate from the processing of clay slurries used to manufacture high voltage ceramic insulators.
- Detecting copper particles in mining operation process steams.
- Monitoring plating bath effluent to help reduce surcharges for wastewater treatment.
- Monitoring microbiological cultures in antibiotics production.
- Making analytical determination of muscle protein extract.
- Monitoring polymer suspension for clarity.

- Assuring optical adhesive clarity in bonding lenses and prisms.
- Detecting the presence of silver chloride that could ruin contacts in circuit board manufacturing (a turbidity check measure).
- Use in turbidity measurement on samples that scale quickly if allowed to cool. (Here, the rapid response of a HACH turbiditmeter makes the difference.).

11

REFRACTOMETER

The identification of properties of substances/ solution by optical method is of special importance in view of the simplicity. The simplest way to identify a solvent using optical methods is to find its refractive index. The term refractive index is defined as follows: when a ray of light travels from one medium to another, there exist a deviation of beam. The ratio of angle of incidence (i) and angle of refraction (r) is called refractive index of one medium relative to another.

$$\frac{\text{Sin } i}{\text{Sin } r} = \frac{n_2}{n_1} \qquad \text{.........} (1)$$

Where n_1 is the refractive index is first medium and n_2 that of second medium. If n_1=1.0 (air) than

$$n_2 = \frac{\text{Sin } i}{\text{Sin } r} \qquad \text{.........} (2)$$

The instrument which uses eq. 2 for determing "n" called as refractometer. Most of the refractometers are designed on the principle of critical angle. The critical angle is defined as the angle of refraction in a medium when radiation is incident on its boundary at grazing or 90°.

$$n_2 = \frac{1}{\text{Sin } r_c}$$

Then where r_c is the critical angle at the wavelength used. If we know either n_1 or n_2, we can find other. In observing phenomenon, the medium 1 is usually the sample and medium 2 a prism of know refractive index 'n'.

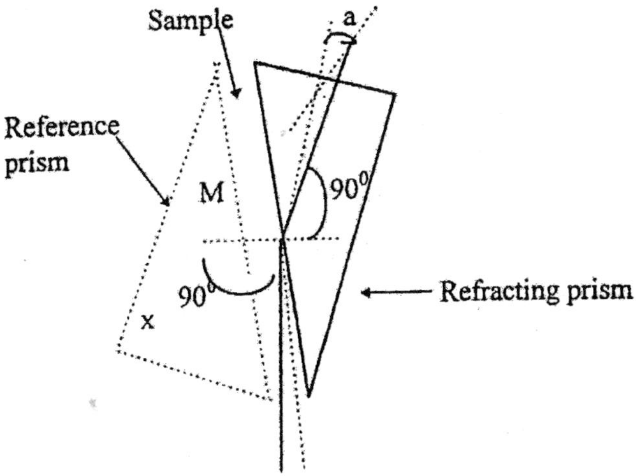

Fig. 1

If the sample is put between two right angle prisms and light is allowed to be incident then all non-grazing rays are refracted at angles smaller that r_c. The dark light boundary is only formed for those rays which are incident at angle 80° - 90°. Since the bandwidth is of 10°, an endless set of parallel critical rays are formed. Condensing lens is therefore, absolutely essential to get single dark-light boundary. In practice, actually 1 to 3 drops of sample liquid are placed between two prisms. The prisms are partially hollowed to allow the circulation of fluid. Light enters through a concave mirror. Next we notice that no substance can be examined having refractive index greater than index of refraction of liquid is greater than R.I. of prism, then only total reflection will be result. Secondly, we do not measure critical angle as it is formed inside prism (See Fig. 1). What is determinable is the angle of emergence of the critical ray. The angle 'α' may be found by scanning the upper edge of refracting prism with a telescope. The prism is so mounted that it pivots about a central point on its surface. When the sharp edge of light-dark boundary has been centered on cross wires of telescope, reading of the index marker is noted. The scale is graduated for yellow line of Na to the nearest 0.001 unit.

In order to achieve cost effectiveness one generally uses tungsten lamp. This being polychromatic introduces chromatic boundary in the telescope. It is compensated by introducing a pair of Amici prisms after refracting prism. With this pair, one can achieve at least no deviation for Na-D-line. This increase the accuracy by 10 %.

PRECISION:

Reliability is increased by a factor of three. More improvements are possible with bigger refracting prisms.

ERROR:

It is cutting of near grazing rays, those incident on refracting prisms at vary small angles. Abbe refracts only the radiation diffused from rough/matte surface of prism into the liquid. Unfortunately, this radiation is poor in grazing rays. As a result of this, true critical boundary is difficult to see. What we see is apparent boundary within shaded region.

90° PRISM:

These are used because, otherwise, loss of intensity would be serious.

Let refractive index of sample be 'n_1' and of prism 'n_2'

$$\frac{n_2}{n_1} = \frac{1}{\text{Sin } r_c}$$

$$\frac{\text{Sin i}}{\text{Sin r}} = n_2$$

$$r + r_c = 90^0$$

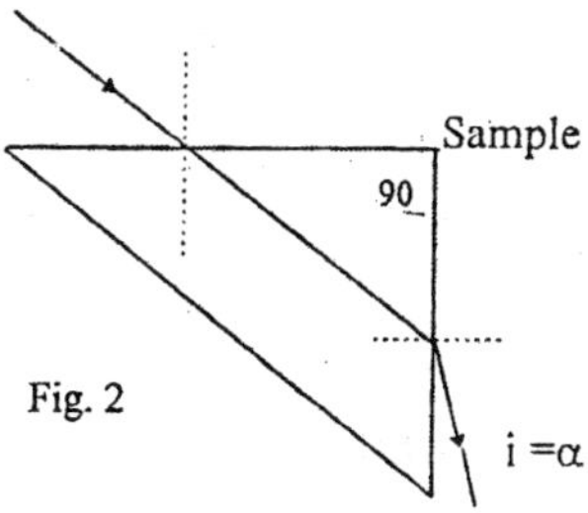

Fig. 2

$$\frac{\text{Sin I}}{\text{Sin}(\pi/2 - r_c)} = \frac{\text{Sin i}}{\text{Sin } r_c} = n2$$

$$\sqrt{1 - \frac{n_1^2}{n_2^2}} = \frac{\text{Sin i}}{n_2} = \frac{\text{Sin } \alpha}{n_2}$$

$$n_1^2 = n_2^2 - \text{Sin}^2 \alpha \quad (n_1 < n_2)$$

IMPORTANCE OF R.I. MEASUREMENTS:

1. Refractive index togather with melting and boiling point is one of the physical constant required in chemical analysis.
2. Few substances have a identical refractive index.
3. n_2 / n_1 = Sini/ Sinr accuracy is available upto six decimals.
4. Uses:
   i. Confirming identify of substance.
   ii. For analysis mixture and process steams.
   iii. For establishing properties of polymers, molecular weight, size and shape.
   iv. Determination of reflectivity and dispersion
   v. 'n' also depends upon wavelength e.g.n =
   vi. 'n' also charges with the pressure of gas
   vii. Knowledge of 'n' helps to determine the orientation of crystal
   viii. For precise observation of 'n', one is required to use monochromatic radiation

ix. 'n' also changes with temperature. Most liquids show 4x10-4 units of charge per 0°C. This necesssitates thermostating of sample.

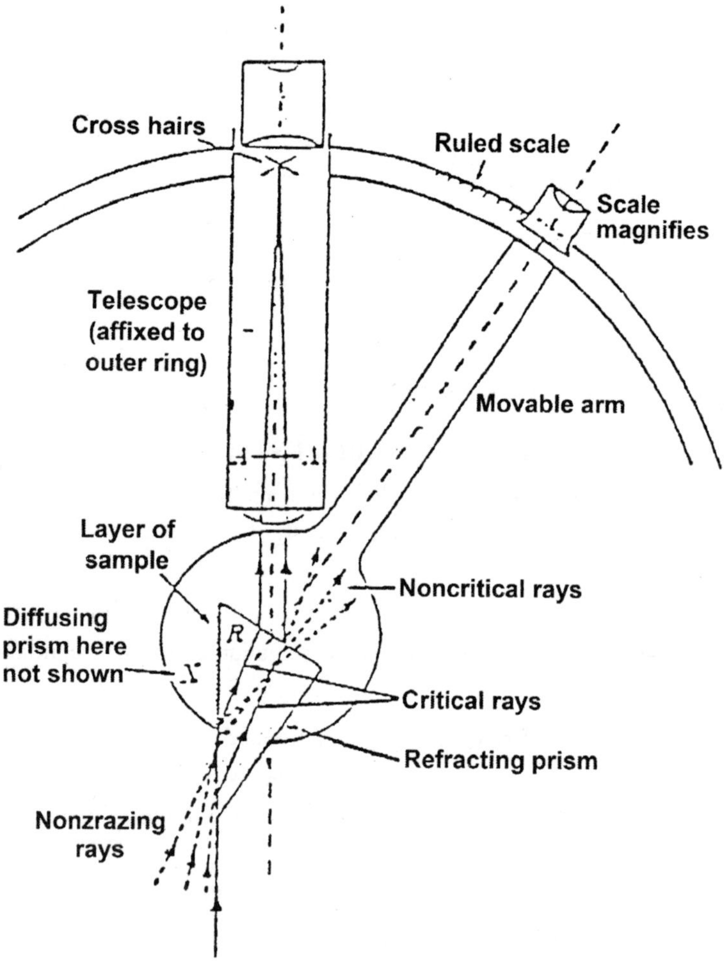

Schematic diagram of an Abbe refractometer. As shown, it is intended for use with chromatic light. To adopt for use white light. Amici prisms may be inserted at AA.

12

POLARIMETER

The identification of some substance is facilitated by eliminating the vibrations of light radiation. The process is referred to as polarisation. When one vibration is eliminated it is called as linearly polarised. A large no. of substances characteristically rotates the plane of polarization. These substances are referred to as optically active e.g. tourmaline crystal which demonstrates that only, transverse vibration of radiation is passed through it while vibration is cut off. This activeness of some substances is due to their structure and due to asymmetric nature.

Optical rotation depends mainly on (a) wavelength (λ) (b) path length (i) (c) temperature (t) (d) density (p) or concentration (c) of the solution. The rotation is measured by a term called as specific rotary power (α)

$$\alpha = 100\ \theta^{\circ} / 1\ wp \text{ --(1)}$$

Where θ, l, w & p are angular rotation of sample in degrees, length in decimeters, of solute in 100 gms of the solution and density of the solution, respectively.

The simple polarimeter consists of following modules.

a. Source
b. Collimator
c. Polariser
d. End point device

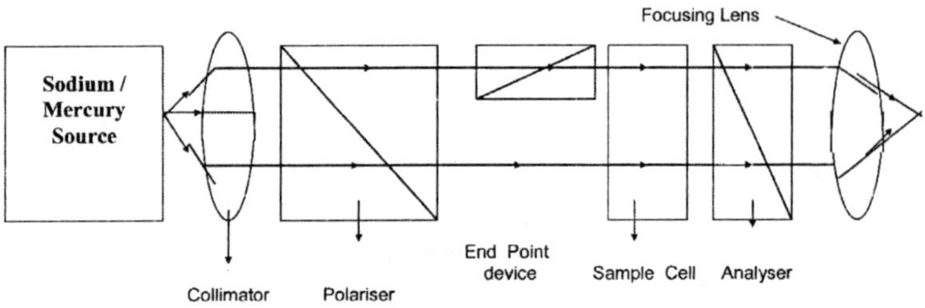

e. Sample Cell

f. Analyser

g. Eye piece

a. Since the specific rotary power has strong dependence on wavelength and varies considerably with each wavelength the source employed is usually monochromatic. The cheapest source is sodium light or mercury lamp with green filter attached to it.

b. The beam from Na/Hg lamp is allowed to fall on collimator. The collimator is an achromatic lens which focusses the beam on polariser.

c. The polariser is a crystal of calcite. This crystal rotates the plane of vibration of radiation. Thus this gives a linearly polarised beam which is now concentrated on end point device.

d.e. Since eye has a poor sensing efficiency for measuring the plane of rotation, it is necessary to alter, the plane of polarisation of 1/2 or 1/3 of the beam energing from polariser. In effect light after passing through end point device splits in two parts one having more intensity and other less. These two beams now falls on sample which further introduces characteristic rotation.

f. After passing through sample, the two light beams passes through analyser made of calcite crystal which further rotates the plane of rotation. When polariser and analyser are at right angles, the intensity is minimum. When analyser is further rotated a half shadow appearance is observed. Note the angle at this stage. The difference in two angular settings gives 'θ'. Thus knowing 'θ', l , w & p one can find 'α'.

13

PH MEASUREMENT

Determination of pH is a very common measurement in laboratories, industry, hospital, soil and water testing and a wide variety of other analytical, control and monitoring operations. Therefore, a large variety of instruments are available commercially for pH measurement, control and monitoring applications. Measurement of pH gives a measure of degree of acidity (or basicity) - concentration of H^+- in a stationary or flowing sample fluid. This is often very crucial in decision making in quality control, process industries, food, beverages and fermentation industry, biological and microbiological operations etc.

Sensing of pH is accomplished by a pH - sensitive glass in contact with the internal fill, a 7 pH buffer, and the external sample. The pH - sensitive glass develops potential as per equations (1) and (3), by proton exchange between H_3O+ in the aqueous solution and in the hydrated gel layer of the glass. The protons enter the sites vacated by Na^+ and recombine with H_3O+ in the hydrated gel layer.

The potential developed is proportional to the difference in logarithms of activity of H_3O+ in solution and in gel layer on both sides of the glass membrane. The log of hydrogen ion activity can be converted to pH using the definition of pH, to give equation (6).

$$E1 = K_9 1 \div 0.1984\,(T + 273.16) \log \frac{a_1}{a_{9^1}} \qquad (1)$$

$$E1 = K_9 1 \div 0.1984\,(T + 273.16)\,[\log a1 - \log a_9 1] \qquad (2)$$

$$E2 = K_9 2 \div 0.1984\,(T + 273.16) \log \frac{a_2}{a_{9^2}} \qquad (3)$$

$$E2 = K_9 2 \div 0.1984\,(T + 273.16)\,[\log a_2 - \log a_{92}] \qquad (4)$$

If $K_9 1 = K_9 2$ and $a_{91} = a_{92}$

$$E_2 - E_1 = 0.1984\,(T + 273.16)\,[\log a_1 - \log a_2] \qquad (5a)$$

$$= 0.1984\,(T + 273.16)\,(pH_2 - pH_1) \qquad (5b)$$

$$= 0.1984\,(T + 273.16)\,(7 - pH_1) \qquad (6)$$

The above series of equations also indicate that:

(1) mV output of electrode decreases as the pH increases

(2) mV output is zero at pH = 7

(3) mV output is +ve below pH 7, and -ve above pH 7.

(4) Effect of temperature on mV output approaches zero as pH approaches 7.

(5) At 25°C, the output changes by 59.16 mV per pH unit (0.1984 x 298.16).

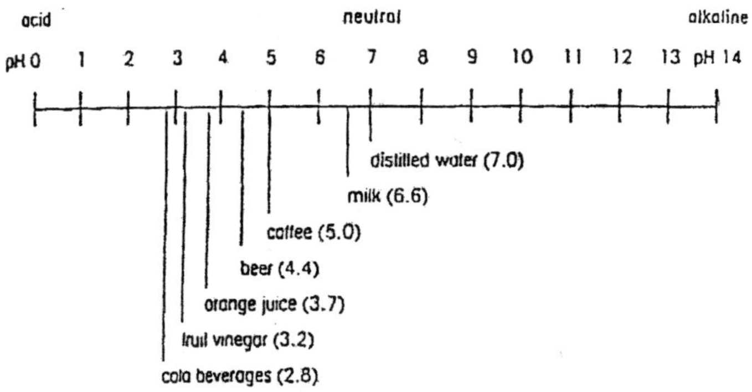

pH values of various food stuffs

Range	pH	H+ concentration (mal/L)	OH- concentration (mal/L)
Acid	0	1	0.00000000000001
	1	0.1	0.0000000000001
	2	0.01	0.000000000001
	3	0.001	0.00000000001
	4	0.0001	0.0000000001
	5	0.00001	0.000000001
	6	0.000001	0.00000001
Neutral	7	0.0000001	0.0000001
Alkaline	8	0.00000001	0.000001
	9	0.000000001	0.00001
	10	0.0000000001	0.0001
	11	0.00000000001	0.001
	12	0.000000000001	0.01
	13	0.0000000000001	0.1
	14	0.00000000000001	1

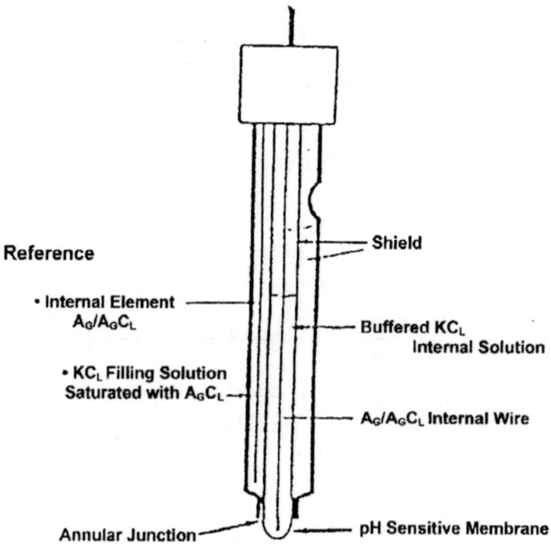

Figure: Combination Electrode

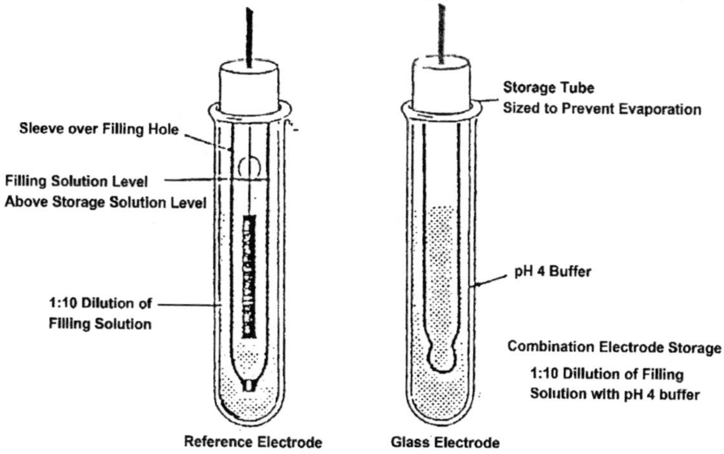

Figure: Electrode Storage

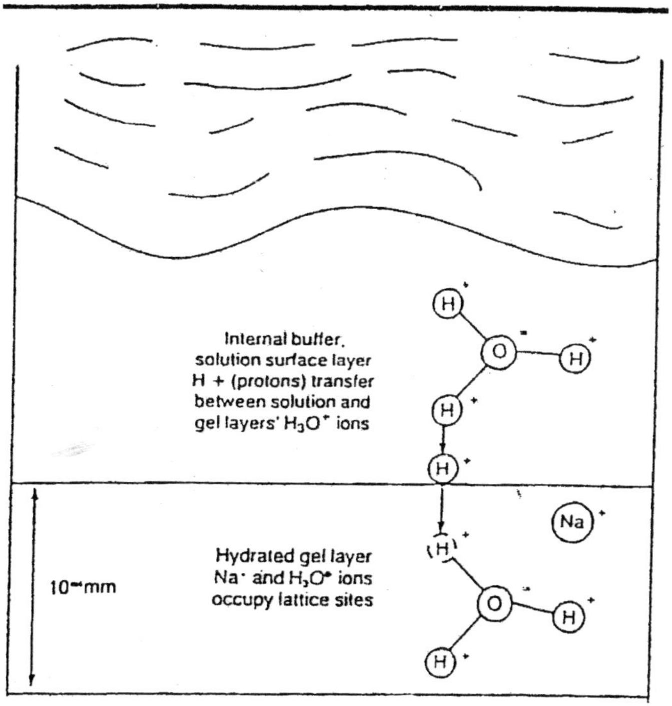

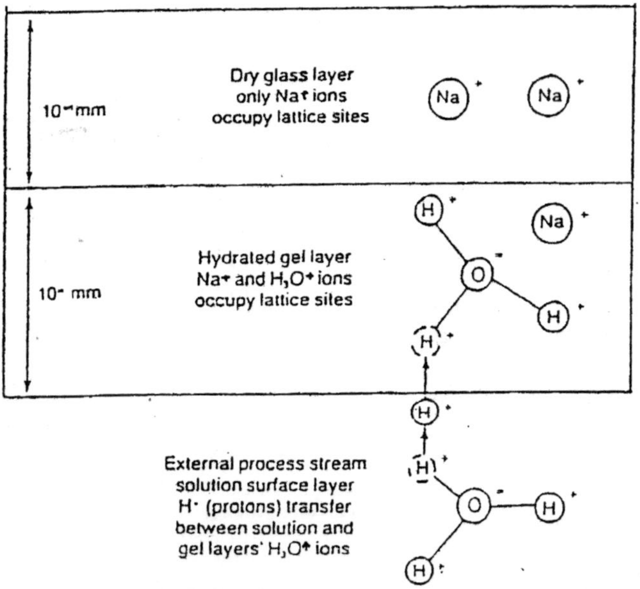

A potential is developed at both the inner and outer glass surfaces of the measurement electrode by proton exchange with a hydrated gel layer.

Type/ Range	Accuracy	High Temp.	ORP	Sodium	Coating	Abrasion	Etching	Cost
Glass Bulb (0 to 14 pH)	+	-	+	+	-	-	-	+
Flat Glass (2 to 12 pH)	+	-	+	-	+	+	-	+
Glass steel (0 to 10 pH)	+	+	+	+	+	+	+	-
Antimony (3 to 11 pH)	-	-	-	-	-	+	+	+
Iridium Oxide (-10 to 20 pH)	+	+	-	+	+	+	+	+
Durafet (0 to 14 pH)	+	+	+	+	+	+	+	+

The ratings of different types of measurement electrodes for various operating conditions. The + denotes a positive or good rating; the - denotes a negative or poor rating.

GLASS ELECTRODES:

A 'gel layer' develops on the pH-sensitive glass membrane when a pH glass electrode comes into contact with an aqueous measuring solution. Such a 'gel layer' arises also on the inside of the glass membrane which is in contact with a defined buffer solution (the inner buffer).

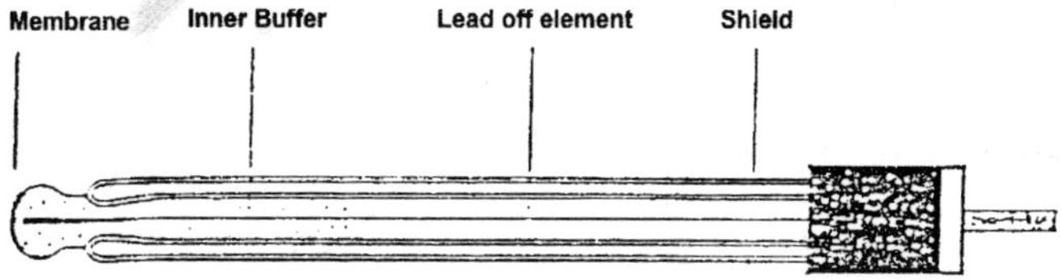

Structure of a glass Electrode

The H^+ ions either diffuse out of the gel layer, or into the gel layer, depending on the pH value of the measured solution. In the case of an alkaline solution the H^+ ions diffuse out and a negative change is established on the outer side of the gel layer. Since the glass electrode has an interact buffer with a constant pH value, the potential of the inner surface of the membrane is also constant during the measurement. The total membrane potential is a result of the difference between the inner and outer change.

$E_{al} = E° - S\,(pHa - pHi)$

E_{al} = Electrode potential

E° = Zero potential

S = Slope (mV per pH unit)

pH1 = Ph value of the internal buffer

pH2 = pH value of the measured solution

Combination Electrodes:

Since the combination electrode (Fig) is much easier to handle than the separate electrode, the former is used almost exclusively today. In the combination electrode the glass electrode is concentrically surrounded by the reference electrolyte.

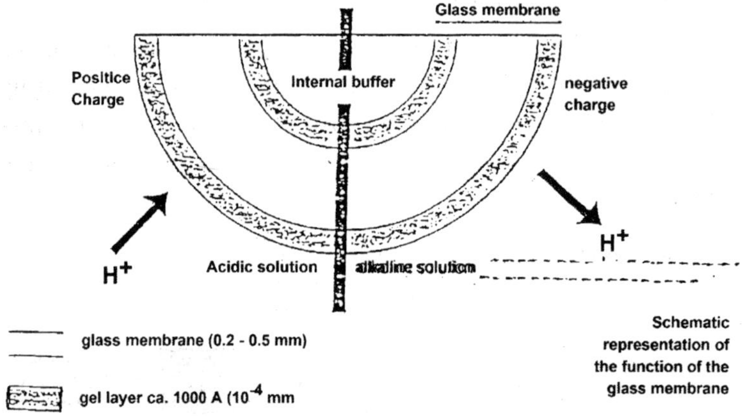

Schematic representation of the function of the glass membrane

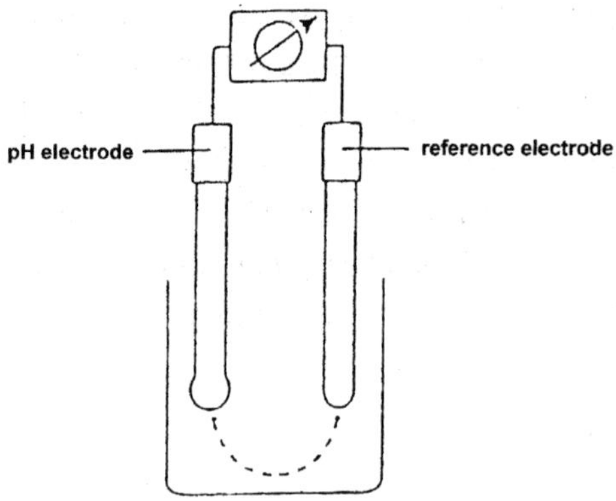

Measuring Circuit

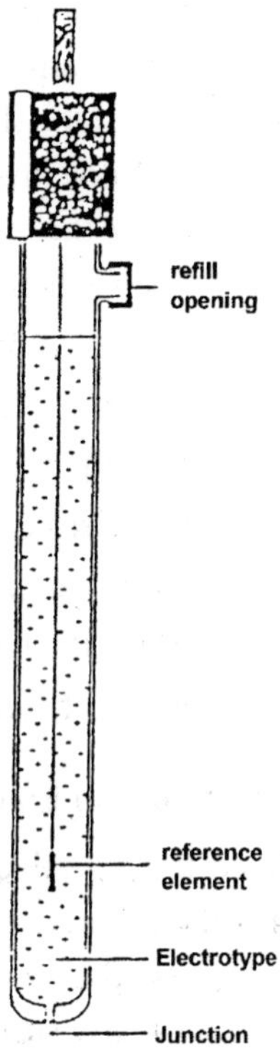

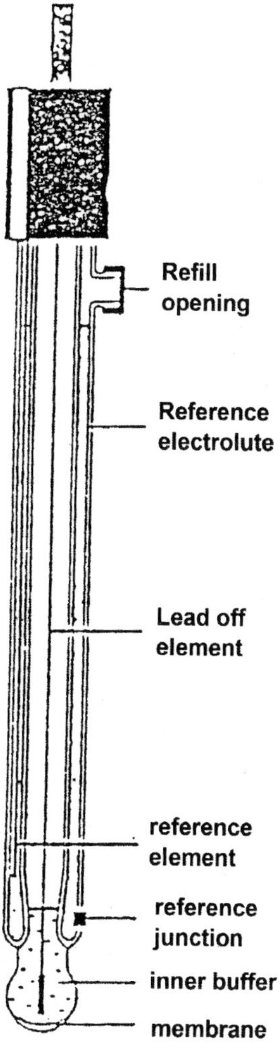

Structure of a Combination electrode

Only when the different parts of the electrode are expected to have very different life expectancies is the use of separate electrodes recommended instead of a single combination electrode.

Three-in-one electrodes:

A recent innovation is the addition of a temperature sensor to the pH combination electrode.

By housing the temperature sensor in the same body as the pH and reference elements, temperature compensated readings can easily be made with a single probe.

PH MEASURING SYSTEM:

Successful pH measurement can only be achieved by choosing the correct system to meet the demands of the sample under examination. As well as the correct apparatus, a supply of suitable reagents is vital.

Consideration has to be given to:

Type of pH meter	Specification, ease of operation
Electrode (S)	Is it suitable for this measurement? Is a pH electrode with built-in temperature senor available?
Temperature probe	Is temperature compensation required?
Buffer solutions	Pure, correct value
Reagents	Distilled water, electrolyte solutions, cleaning solutions
Glassware	Clean labelled
Electrode holder	For housing electrode (S)

PH ELECTRODE SYSTEMS:

Troubleshooting guide:

The first important step in troubleshooting is to isolate the problem to one of the six major elements of the pH measuring system, which are:

pH meter	Buffer Solution
pH electrode	Operator
Reference electrode	Application

Once this is done, action can be taken to correct the problem:

pH Meters:

Symptoms usually related to pH failure are offscale readings that will not change. To confirm that the meter is the source of the problem, refer to the instruction manual accompanying the meter.

Electrodes:

There are three types of electrode used in the determination of pH:

(i) Reference Electrodes

(ii) pH Electrodes

(iii) Combination electrodes (pH and reference electrode in one sensor)

ELECTRODE TYPES

Reference Electrode

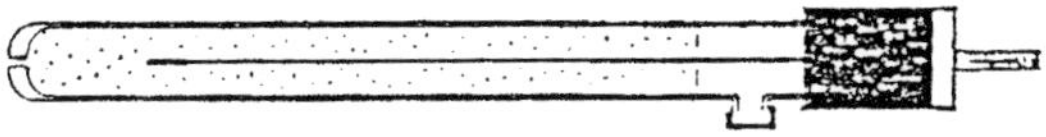

pH electrode

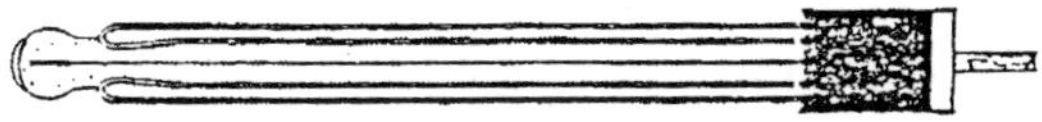

Combination Electrode

ELECTRODE STORAGE:

(i) Reference Electrodes:

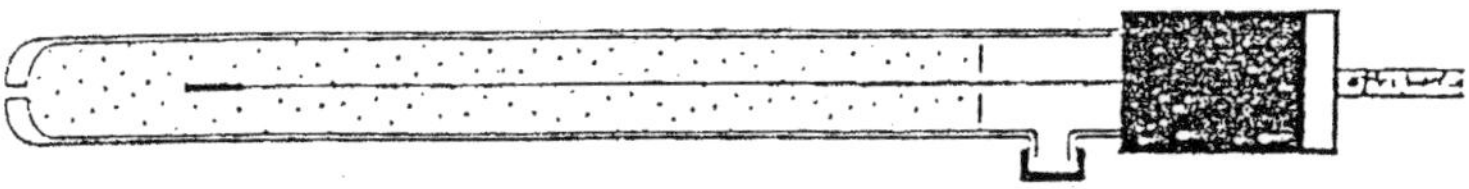

Short term	Long term
Immerse in reference Filling solution.	Store with wetting cap attached filled with Reference filling solution. Close side aperture.

(ii) pH Electrodes:

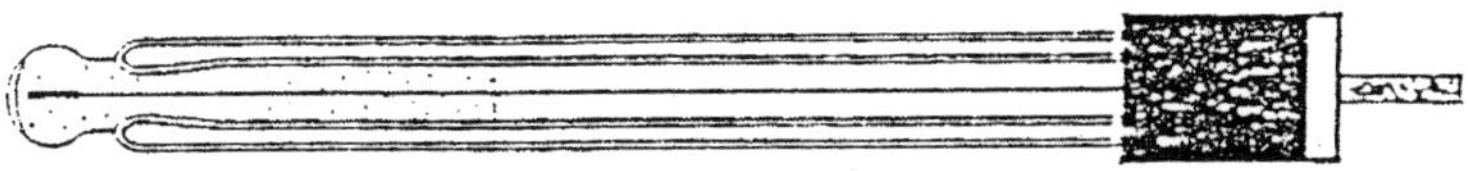

Short term	Long term
Immerse in reference Filling solution.	Store with wetting cap attached filled with Reference filling solution.

(iii) Combination electrodes:

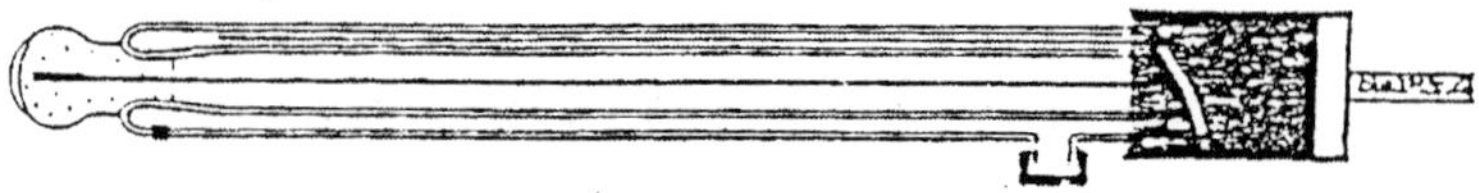

Short term	Long term
Immerse in filling	Store with wetting cap attached
Reference solution.	Containing reference filling solution.
	Close side aperture.

Fig. 16: Electrode Storage

Directly after use and before a period of storage the electrodes should be rinsed thoroughly with distilled water.

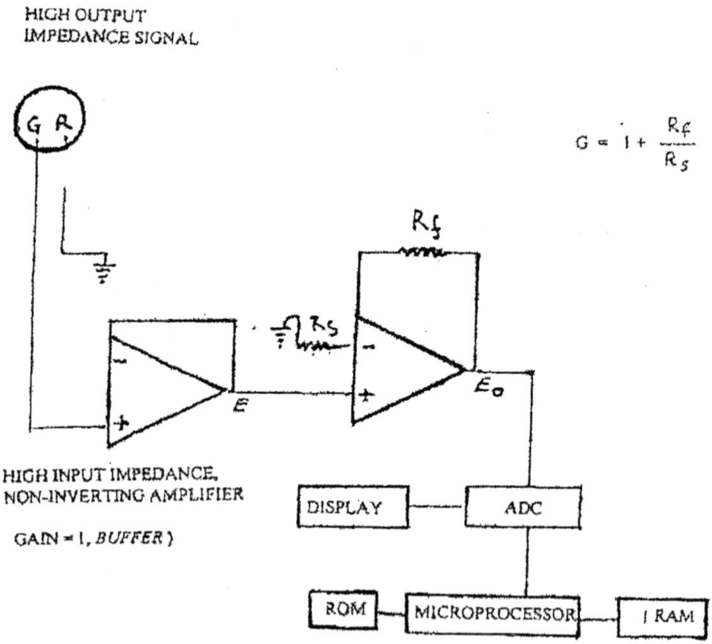

MICROPROCESSOR - BASED pH METER
(With out Temperature Compensation)

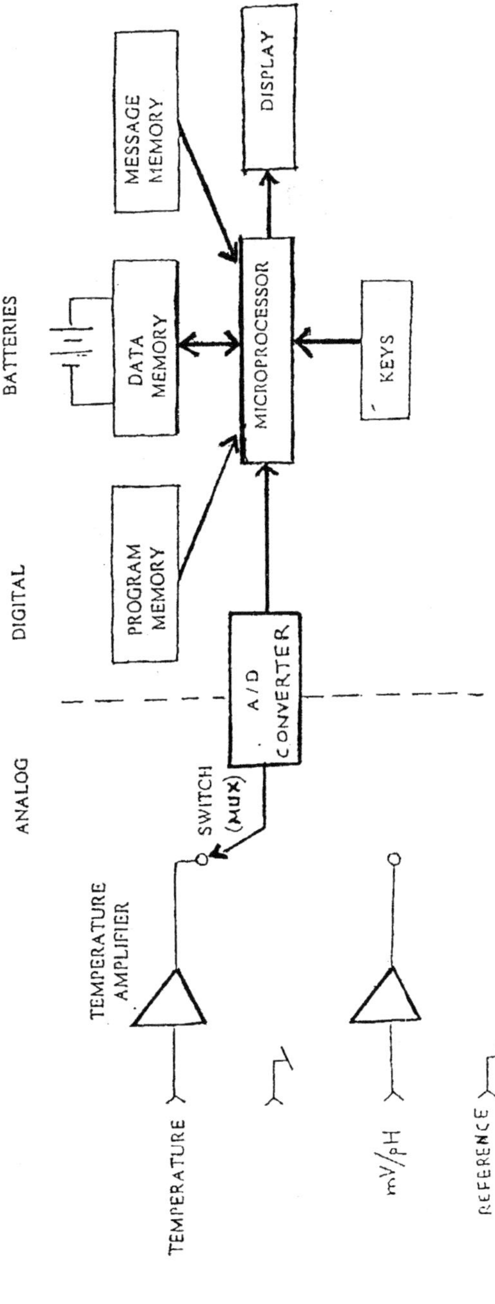

MICROPROCESSOR - BASED pH METER
(With Temperature Compensation)

14

CONDUCTIVITY MEASUREMENT

Dissolved solids and dissolved gases confer varying degree of electrolytic conductance on aqueous solutions. Measurement of conductivity provides information about the total ionic content of a solution. It is non-specific. This, however, can be used with advantage to characterize the purity of potable waters and monitoring effectiveness of water demineralisers. Conductance can be used effectively to measure concentration of acids, bases and certain solutes which give monotonic, and in some cases even linear, conductance-concentration plot over wide concentration ranges. Since electrolytes vary with respect to their ability to conduct current, conductance measurements provide a valuable method of analyzing binary mixtures of electrolytes. Conductor metric titrimetry is a useful method for following the course of reactions involving electrolytes. Conductivity sensors with suitably modified design have found applications in process control instrumentation. Finally, electrical conductivity detectors find useful role in modern Ion Chromatographic and HPLC instrumentation.

The electrical conductance is the reciprocal of the resistance, usually given the symbol L, with units of siemens (S) or reciprocal ohms (mhos, Ω^{-1}). The resistance of a sample is property of its geometry– its cross-sectional area A and its length L for our purpose, the area is usually taken as the area of each of pair of parallel electrodes, and the length L of the sample is replaced by d, the distance between them. The specific resistance (resistively), denoted by *P*, has the units of ohm-cm and it is defined by *P* = R (A/d). Similarly, the specific conductance or conductivity is denoted by the symbol k with the units of siemens per cm, so that

$$K = 1/P\,(1/R)\,(d/A) = L\,\theta$$

Where θ is equal to d/A in cm^{-1}. Since θ is function only of the geometry of the measuring electrodes, its is useful in characterization of cells, and hence is called the cell constant. Cell constants can be determined by measurement of solutions of known specific conductance.

Table1. Reference Solutions for Calibration of ceil Constants.

Approx. Molars	Method of frequenron	Temp. (°C)	L (µS/cm)
		0	65.176
1.0	74.2460 g. KCL per litre of solution at 20°C	18	97.838
		25	111.342
		0	7.138
0.1	7.4365 g. KCL per litre of solution at 20°C	18	11.167
		25	12.856
		0	773.6
0.01	0.7440 g. KCL per litre of solution at 20°C	18	1.220.5
		25	1.408.8
0.001	Dilute 100 ml. of 0.01M to 1 litre at 20°C	25	146.93

Electrolutic Theory:

Since the conductance is determined by the totality of ions present in a solution, largely acting independently of each other, it can be expressed as a summation.

$$L = 10^{-3}\,\theta^{-1}\,\Sigma\, z_i c_i \lambda_i$$

in which c_i represents the molar concentration of the ith ion, z_i its charge, and λ_i its equivalent ionic conductivity. The summation covers all ions of both signs. Molar conductivity, is sometimes defined as $\lambda = \lambda + \lambda - = 1000$ k/C. Its units are S.cm^2 mo^{-1}. The quantity λ is a property of ions (either positive or negative) that gives quantitative information about their relative contribution to the conductance of the solution. Its value is to some extent dependent on the total ionic concentration, increasing with increasing dilution. Representative numerical values of λo the limiting value λ of as the concentration approaches zero (infinite dilution), are given below.

Useful information pertaining to ionic equilibria can be obtained from conduct O$^-$ metric data, particularly where ions tend

Table 2: Equivalent Ionic Conductivity of selected Ions Infinite Dilution in S cm2 m at 25°c

Cations (a)	λΩ	Terapco (b)	Anions (a)	λΩ	Terapco (b)
H^+	349.5	0.0139	OH	109.6	0.018
$Co(NH_3)_6^{3+}$	102.3	--	Fe $(CN)_6^{1-}$	110.5	0.02
K^+	73.5	0.0193	Fe $(CN)_6^{3-}$	101.0	--
NH_4^+	73.5	0.019	Co $(CN)_6^{3-}$	98.9	--
Pb^{2+}	69.46	0.02	So_4^{2-}	80.0	0.022
La^{3+}	69.6	0.023	Br^-	78.40	0.0198
Fe^{3+}	68.0	--	I^-	76.8	0.197
Ba^{2+}	63.64	0.023	Cl^-	76.4	0.0202
Ag^+	61.9	0.021	$C_2O_4^{2-}$	74.2	0.02
Ca^{2+}	59.50	0.0230	NO_3^-	71.42	0.020
Cu^{2+}	53.6	0.02	CO_3^{2-}	69.3	0.02
Fe^+	54.0	--	CO_4^-	67.3	0.020
Mg^{2+}	53.06	0.022	HCO_3^-	44.5	--
Zn^{2+}	52.8	0.02	$CH_3CO_2^-$	40.9	0.022
Na^+	50.11	0.0220	$HC_2O_4^-$	40.2	--
Li^+	33.69	0.0235	$C_6H_5CO_2^-$	32.4	0.023
$(n\text{-}Bu)_4N^+$	19.5	0.02	Picrate	30.4	0.025

(a) For ions of change the figure given are on an equivalent basis, so that they apply to the fraction (1/z) of a mole. (b) The temperature coefficient when known, is gives as $(1/\lambda_0)$ (dλaT) with the units of K^{-1}

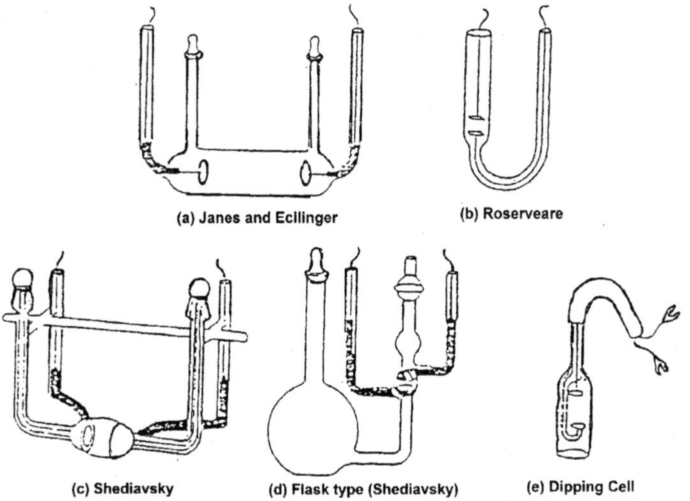

Fig. 1: A selection of cells for measurement of conductance. (a) The form most used for exacting physicochemical measurements. (b) The Roseveare cell is easy to make with the cameras of square pieces of platinum sealed into the glass walls. (c) This form has conical electrodes. Useful for liquids that have a tendency to foam. (d) A flask form convenient for preparing and measuring very dilute solutions. (e) The dipping cell widely used for routine measurements. (From Daniels, F. Alberty, R.A. Williams, J.W., Cornwell, C.D., Bender, P., and Hariman, J.E. Experimental Physical Chemistry, 7th Ed. McGraw-Hill, New York, 1970, with permission)

to be removed form solution by an equilibrium process. Examples:- combination of anions with hydrogen cation to from partially dissociated molecular acids; formation of complexes between metallic cations and various ligands; formation of sparingly soluble salts, etc. Thus measurement of conductance can lead to determination of acidic and basic dissociation constants, stability constants and solubility product constants.

INSTRUMENTATION:

There are two general types of devices for measuring conductance. The first, and most widely used employs a pair of contacting

Table 3: Recommended Cell Constants for various Conductance Ranges.

Conductance Ranges (μS/cm)	Cell Constant (cm^{-1})
0.05 – 20	0.01
1 – 200	0.1
10 – 2000	1.0
100 – 20,000	10.0
1000 – 200,000	50.0

electrodes, frequently platinum, immersed in the test liquid; whereas the second depends upon inductive or capacitive effects to measure the conductance.

IMMERSED ELECTRODE MEASUREMENTS:

Two Electrode Cells: Fig. 1 shows some types of conductivity cells available commercially. Some of them are for precision physico-chemical measurements, others beings more convenient for routine use. Cells with cell constants of 1.0 and 0.1 are the most widely used. The electrodes are usually fabricated from platinum, though graphite, uranium and tungsten are occasionally used. Pt electrodes are coated with a finely divided form the metal (platinum black) platinised platinum. This coating is produced in situ by a few minutes of electrolysis in a solution of chloroplatinic acid containing a small amount of lead acetate. The electrolysis should be repeated with reversed polarity. After Platinizing, the electrodes should be stored in distilled water.

CONDUCTIVITY METERS FOR TWO-ELECTRODE CELLS:

Two-electrode cells can be used with many commercially available instruments. The oldest principle of Wheatstone bridge is still found in a number of instruments for reasons of simplicity and universal usage. A disadvantage, however, is the need to adjust the bridge manually. Fig 2 illustrates such a bridge.

Modified Wheatstone bridges are among the most precise instruments. The bridge principle can be used for direct-reading

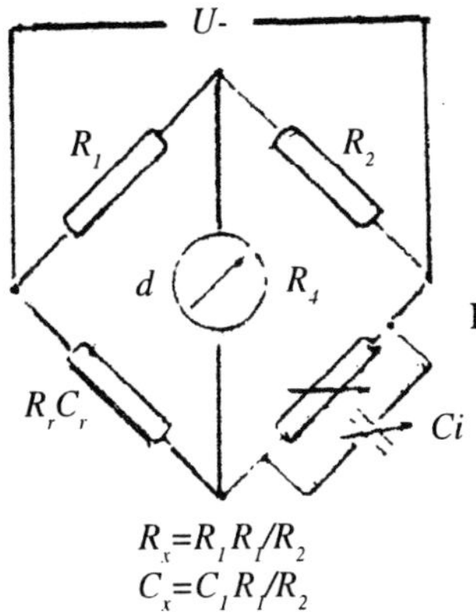

Fig. 2: **Simplified circuit of a Wheatstone bridge to measure the resistance R of two-electrode cells. The cell has to be runed manually with the help of R and R to the minium of the meter J.**

instruments, as shown in Fig. 3. The best means of obtaining a linear response is to use operational amplifiers as in Fig. 4. A box diagram of the circuit of a complete conductivity meter is shown in Fig. 5. Means for automatic temperature compensation are standard in all industrial and precise laboratory applications.

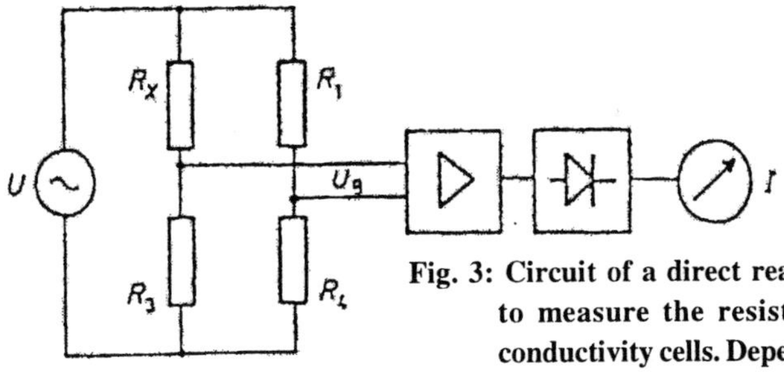

Fig. 3: **Circuit of a direct reading bridge to measure the resistance Rx of conductivity cells. Depending on the ratio R_3/Rx the read-out of I is nearly linear or logarithmic.**

Fig.4: **Circuit of a conductivity meter using an operational amplifier with a feedback resistor R_F. The reading I of the meter is linearly proportional to the conductance Gx.**

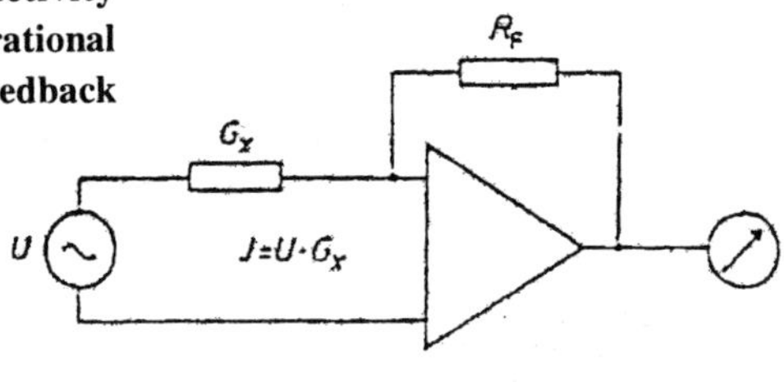

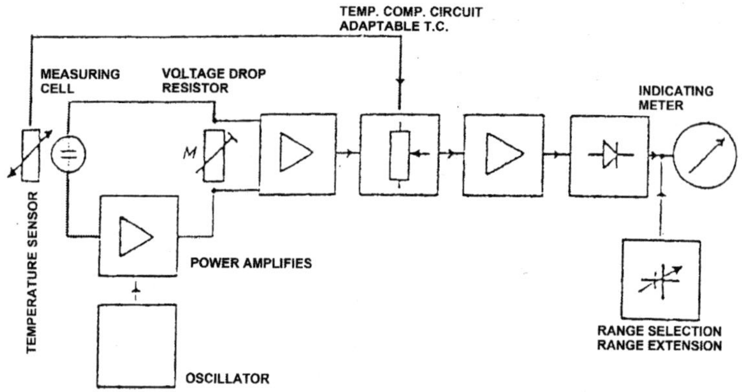

Fig. 5: Detailed circuit of an industrial conductivity meter using the voltage drop principle. The current in the circuit containing the measuring cells causes a voltage drop across the standard resistance M. By changing M the range can be selected. With the help of a temperature sensor automatic compensation of temperature effects can be achieved.

Generally, for all two electrode cells it is postulated that their resistance Rx in contact with a sample should be kept within the limits of $100\ \Omega < Rx < 100\ k\ \Omega$. This can be achieved only with a range of cell constants from 10 - 2 to 10 cm-1. Such cells make use of a different construction to that of the two-electrode concept. Some of the commercially available cells are illustrated in Fig.6-8. The construction in Fig. 8 is unusual. The field lines of the electric field which penetrate the sample are entirely in homogeneously distributed. As a result, the cell has fixed constant only within a limited range of conductivities. Its advantage is, however, that is insensitive to air and/or gas bubbles in the sample.

Practical realization of two-electrode cell is illustrated in Fig.9. However, the concept of conductivity cells need more careful handing since the resistance of the cell is included in a network of other resistances and capacitances. The equivalent circuit of two-electrode cells is shown in Fig.10. C_3 is the capacity of the cable from the cell to the amplifier. In industrial applications it is of the

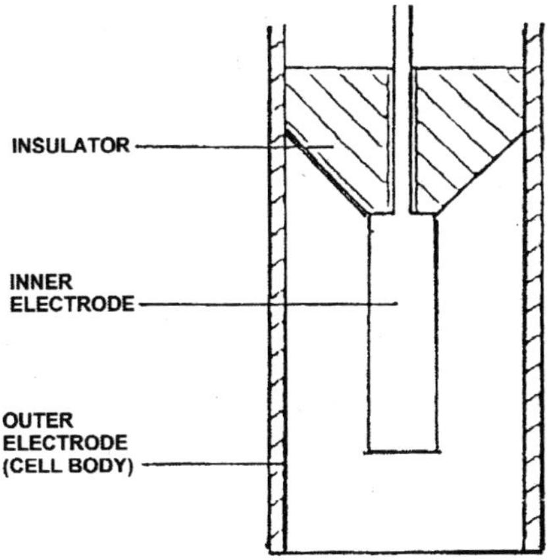

Fig. 6: Two-electrode cell with concentric electrode arrangement. The cell is free of shunt effects

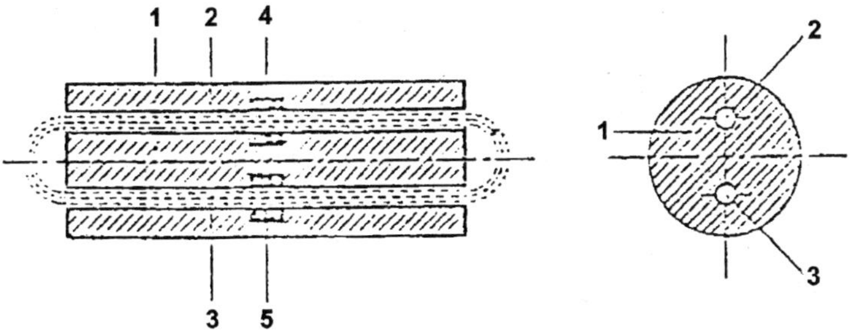

Fig. 7: Two-electrode cell based on the principle of a "long current path" to achieve large values of the cell constants k (upto k = 100 cm) (1) Cell body; (2), (3) Channels filled with the sample; (4), (5) electrodes.

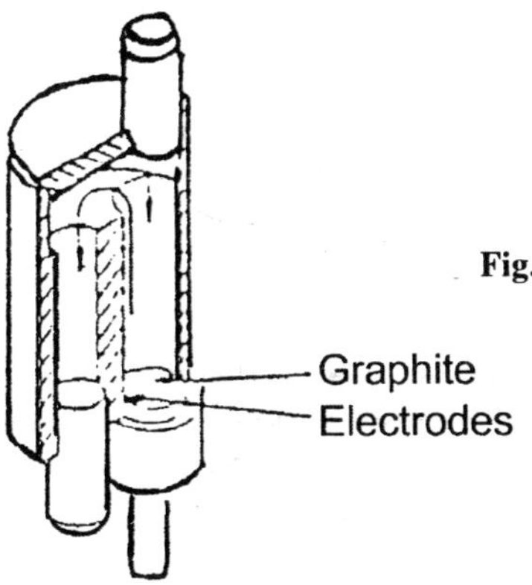

Fig. 8: Two-electrode cell with a heterogeneous field distributions. The arrows indicate the sample flow. Cells of this type are insensitive to bubbles and particles in the sample (WTW)

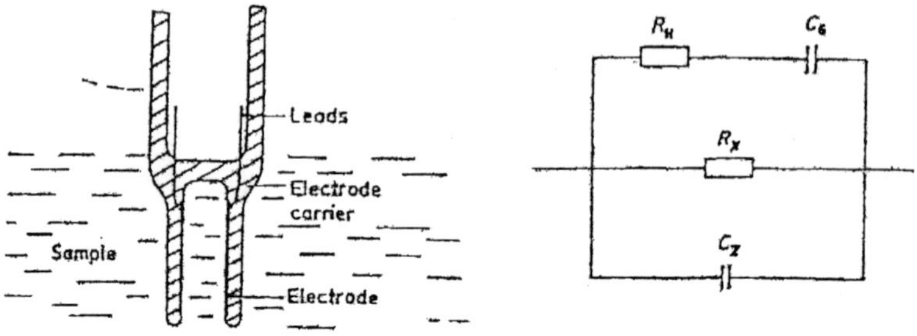

Fig. 9: Practical realization of a two-electrode cell. At higher frequencies shunt effects can be observed via the glassy electrode carrier (C_G) and the resistance (R_H) within the solution.

order of 100 pF/m. R_4 and C_4 are strongly dependent on the construction of the cell. Both components are part of a shunting circuit which will be observed, for instance, in call made in accordance with Fig.9. The contribution of R_4 and C_4 is, however, negligible in concentric cell construction principle shown in Fig.7. The other components within the rectangle surrounded by a dashed line are part of electrode reactions to be found at the interfaces of the electrodes with the samples.

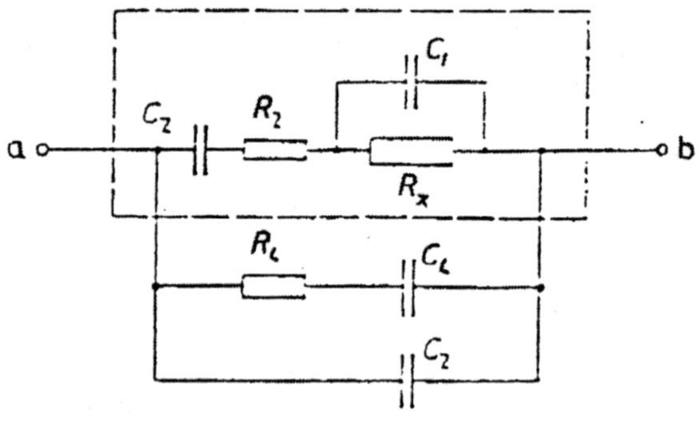

Fig.10: Equivalent circuit of a two electrode cell. The resistance of interest, Rx is part of a multi-component network of other resistors and capacitors. The dashed line rectangle includes all components deriving form electrode reaction; the others are caused by connections and cables.

MULTI-ELECTRODE CELLS:

The main disadvantage of two-electrode cells is that any physical and/or electrochemical change in the electrodes directly influence the results. This is true for all of the effects considered as polarization, for electrode corrosion by chemically aggressive solutions, and for the spoiling of the electrodes, e.g. by oil film or precipitates. To overcome these disadvantage, cells have been developed in recent years which utilize at least four electrodes. In the simplest case two of the electrodes are connected to a constant voltage source which results in the flow of constant current I. Within the field generated by case "current electrodes" another two "voltage electrodes" are placed. They measure the voltage drop U=I. Rx by means of a high-impedance amplifier. In Fig.11, an internal control loop maintains a constant voltage drop U across the voltage electrodes. To achieve this, the current has to be controlled so that it is proportional to the conductivity.

Fig.12 show the principle of measurements in which the current-carrying outer electrodes function similarly to the two-electrode cell in which the measured resistance depends, not only on the solution, but also the resistance of any coatings that might develop on the electrodes. Ohm's law is given for this situation by E = I (R solution - R coating), where E is the voltage across, and I the current through, the electrodes. Thus, with the two-electrode circuit, the measured resistances (or its reciprocal, the conductance) is the sum of the solution and coating resistances. However, the resistance of the electrode coating does not affect EVME, the measured voltage between the inner electrodes, because no current is drawn through them. With an independently measured value of the current, I. through the current-carrying electrodes, the resistance of the solution can be calculated from the following equation and the potentiometrically measured voltage.

Rsolution = Evme / I

It is essential for both two-and four- electrode cells, that the source voltage must be AC supply, since direct current could cause unwanted electrochemical reactions and polarization at the electrodes.

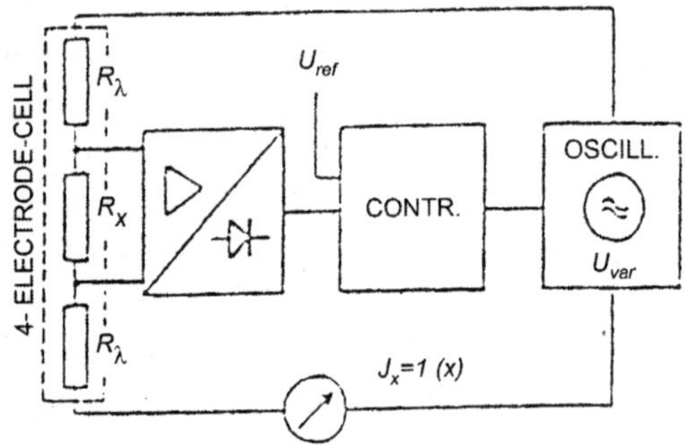

Fig.11: Four-electrode conductivity meter...A controller circuit compares a preselected voltage Uvef with the voltage drop across the resistance Rx Any deviation will be compensated by a variation Uvar of the oscillator. The current Im depends linearly on the conductivity of the sample.

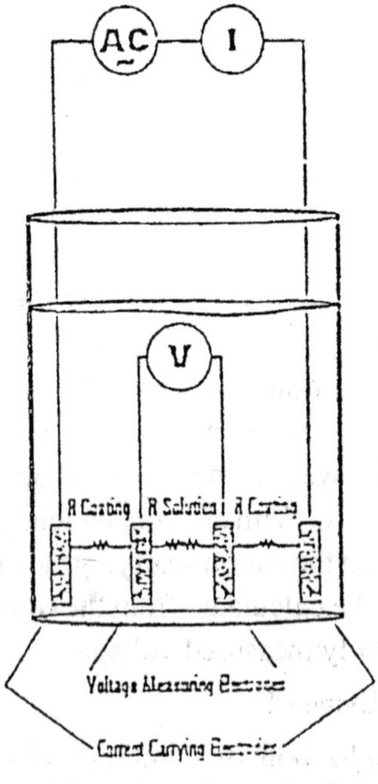

Fig.12: Principle of four-electrode conductivity measurements

CONTACTLESS CELLS:

For electrochemical electrode reactions, cells with direct contact of the electrodes to the conducing solutions can only be a compromise. A different situation, however, can be expected for contactless cells. Several types of contactless cells have been developed which use two entirely different concepts - inductive and capacitive.

INDUCTIVE CONDUCTIVITY CELLS:

Inductive contactless cells were introduced independently by Calvert and Solomon in 1958. The concept is simple. Two coils of a transformer are magnetically shielded form each, other; the only coupling loop is formed by a non-metallic and non-conducting tube which is filled with the sample. Fig.13 illustrates the principle. The voltage induced in the secondary coil depends only on the input voltage of the primary coil and the conductance G of the sample. Typical working frequencies are from 50 to 500 Hz. The entire ranges of conductivities of practical interest can be covered by one cell. By selecting organic polymers as the cell body, a high degree of chemical resistance can by achieved. This, however, imposes a limitation on the admissible temperatures and pressures. Fig. 14 shows a typical example of such a cell.

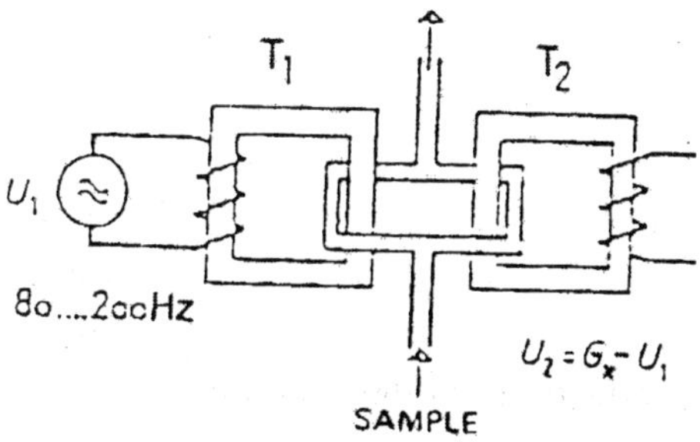

Fig.13: Principle of an inductive contactless conductivity cell. The two halves T_1 and T_2 of a transformer are magnetically shielded from each other. The only coupling between the two coils is achieved by a loop of a non-conducting material which is filled with the sample. The output voltage U_2 depends linearly on the conductance Gx.

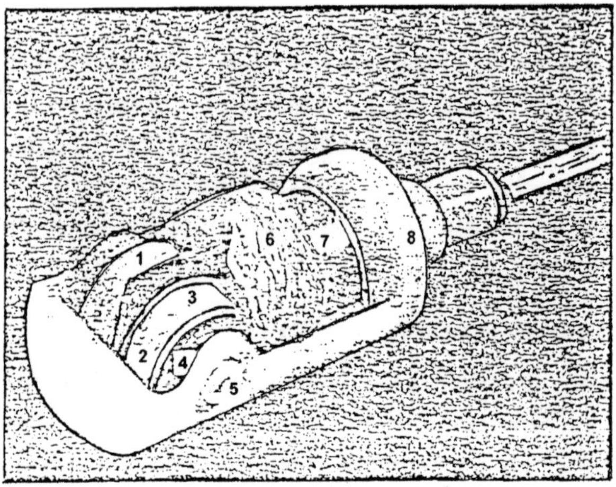

Fig.14: Section through an inductive contactless conductivity cell. 1, 3 Two halves of a transformer with a magnetic shield between; 2, 2 primary/ secondary coil; 4 ring-shaped temperature sensor for automatic temperature compensation; 5-smaple channel; 6-thermal insulation; 7- preamplifier; 8-cell body made of Tefzel

The low frequency method (20-50 kHz) of electrodeless conductivity, often called 'inductive conductivity', has become popular, especially in chemical process and industrial solution applications. The system utilizes a probes consisting of two encapsulated toroids in close proximity to each other, as shown in Fig.15. One toroid generates an alternating electric field in the solution, while the other acts as the receiver to pick up a signal from the field. The equivalent circuit may be compared to a transformer with the toroids forming the primary and secondary windings, as seen in Fig. 16. The transformer core consists of the solution itself. The efficiency with which alternating current is transferred form the primary to the secondary depends on the conductivity of the solution.

Several configurations are possible. One, designed for immersion, is shown in Fig.17. The toroids are covered with a chemically resistant fluorocarbon or other high temperature thermoplastic material. Any precipitates or coatings adhering to the probe generally have little or no effects on the measured conductance. A configuration in which the probe does not come in contact with the solution is shown in Fig.18. The toroid unit is installed around a section of non conducting pipe containing the test solution. A complete liquid loop must exist for this arrangement to work.

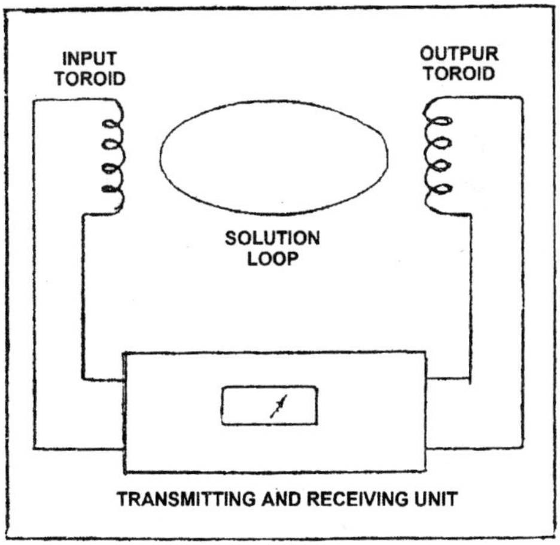

Fig.15: The principle of the electrodeless conductivity cell and instrument (Foxboro)

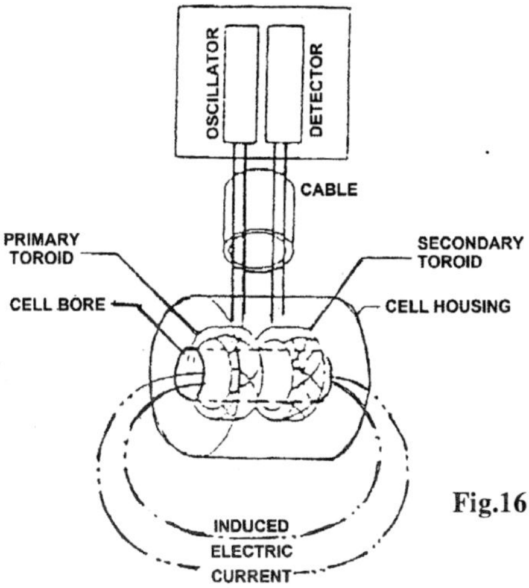

Fig.16: Simplified representation of an electrodeless conductivity measuring circuit.

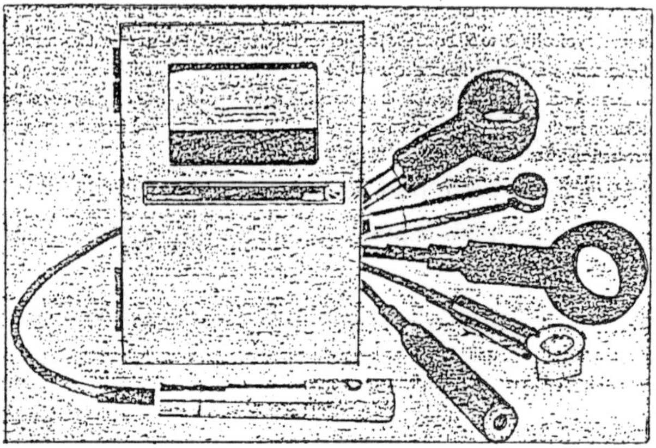

Fig.17: An electrodeless conductivity instrument with an assortment of cells (Foxboro).

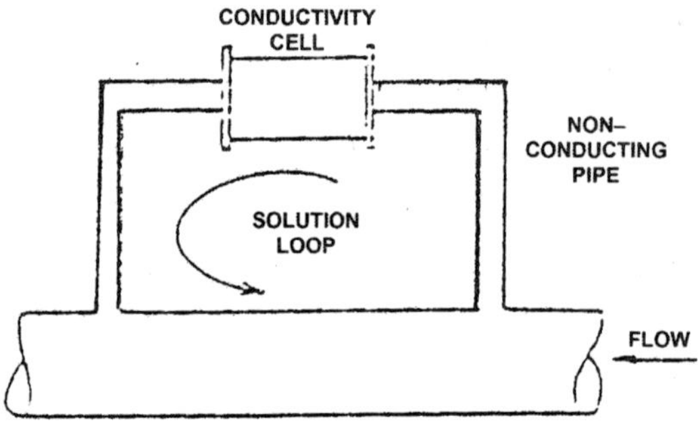

Fig.18: An electrodeless conductivity cell mounted externally to a segment of glass or plastic pipe forming a solution loop in an industrial flow line.

The generating toroid is energized from a stable audio-frequency source, typically 20-50 kHz. The pick-up toroid is connected to a receiver that measures the current through this secondary winding. The current is then amplified and sent to an analog recorder or to a computer. The current is a direct function of the conductance of the solution in the loop, in a manner completely analogous to the conventional measurement with contacting electrodes. The useful range of instruments extends from 0-100 μS/cm to 0-2 S/cm, with relative accuracy of a few tenth of a percent of FSD, after temperature compensation. A temperature sensor is incorporated into the toroid probe, and compensation circuit corrects all reading to the standard reference temperature of 25°C.

Such instruments are manufactured commercially for analysis and control in chemical process industries and in other continuous monitoring applications. Although its stability, accuracy, and freedom from maintenance are superior to contacting conductivity techniques, lack of bench models has hindered its laboratory use and applications. The smallest electrodelss probe in about 3.6 cm in diameter, has a constant of 2.5 cm^{-1}, and requires a minimum solution volume of several hundred milliliters to ensure a complete solution loop without wall effects which distort the apparent cell constant. For the lower conductance ranges, which require a smaller cell constant, the diameter of the probe must be increased, and accurate measurement below about 10 μS/cm is not practical.

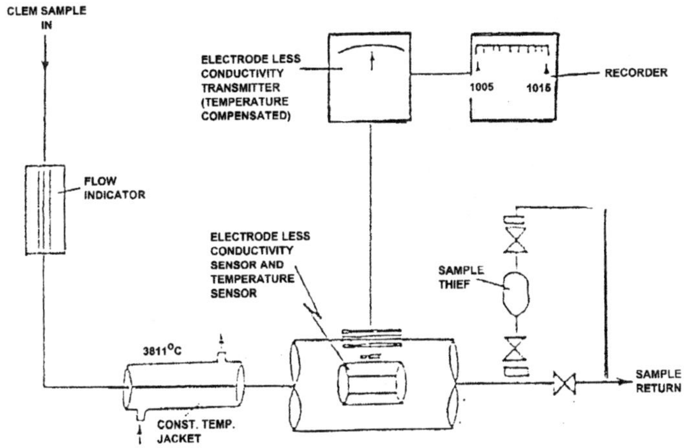

Fig.19: A continuous analyzer for oleum (fuming sulphuric acid), using an electrodeless conductivity cell. The sample thief collects a titratable sample, unaffected by atmospheric moisture, which is used in instrument calibration.

Numerous applications of electrodeless conductivity have been recommended for the chemical, pulp and paper, aluminium, mining, and food industries. An instrument for the continuous analysis of oleum in the range of 100-102 percent equivalent suphuric acid, with an accuracy of 0.01% is shown in Fig.19.

The principle underlying this technique is entirely different from the foregoing. As shown in Fig. 20, two-ring shaped electrodes are placed on the outside of a non-conducting cell body. A high frequency voltage of the order of 1-100 MHz is applied across these electrodes. A finite part of the electric field penetrates the internal core section of the cell body, which is filled with the conducting sample.

The equivalent circuit of such a cell is also shown in the Figure. Depending upon the frequency and/or the conductance, the cell can be treated as a conductance Gres, or a capacill Gres. Each of the equations contains the cell parameters Cs and Cp, and in the letter a contribution of the dielectric constant ε of the solution is included:

$$Cres = G_2 G_3 + w^2 Cs\ Cp^2 + w^2 Cs^2 Cp/G_2 \div 2\ (Cs \div Cp)^2$$

$$Cres = Gw^2 Cs/G^2 + w^2 (Cs + Cp)^2$$

Where Cp = εCo, and Co is the vacuum capacity of the cell. As expected, the response characteristic derived using these equations are far from linear, as confirmed in Fig.21. The dynamic range of the Cres plot covers three decades of conductance whilst the Gres values pass through a maximum. Despite these serious disadvantages of capacitive cells, much experimental work has been carried out, which in most instances was related to the end-point detection of "high-frequency" titrations.

APPLICATIONS:

Conductmetric titrimetry is widely applicable for titration reactions involving ions. Fig. 22 indicates the kind of curves that result in the titration of acids of various dissociation constants with sodium

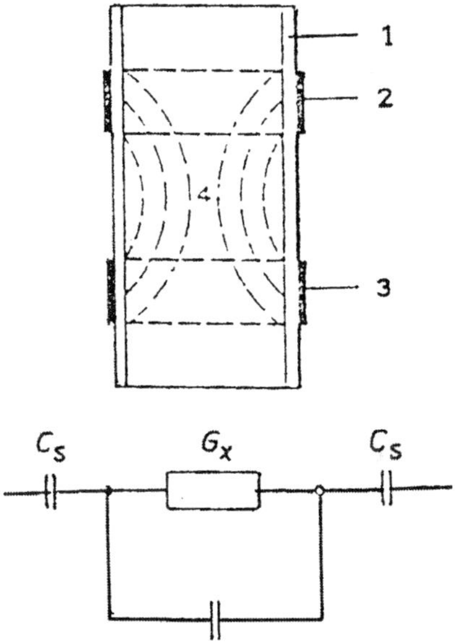

Fig.20: Non-metallic and non-conducting cell body; 2.3 Ring-shaped electrodes on the outside body; 4 sample volume penetrated by high frequency field. The equivalent circuit shows to capacitances Cs which are caused by the conducting electrodes, the cell body (= dielectric) and the conducting sample. Cp contains a contribution of the dielectric constant of the sample solution. Gx is the conducatance of the sample.

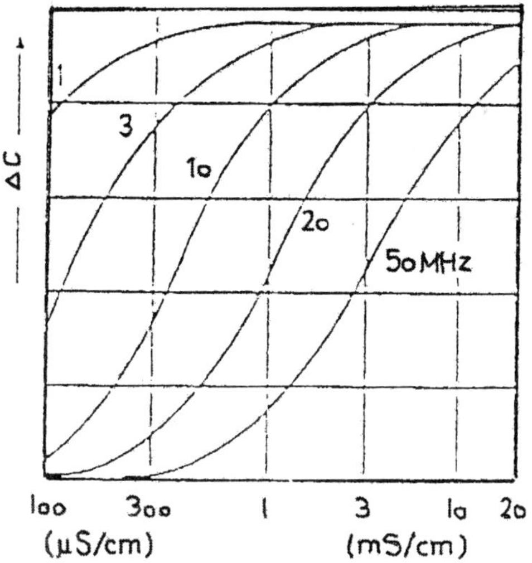

Fig.21: Response characteristic of a capacitive contanctless conductivity cell using the resulting capacity Cres. The range of optimum sensitivity can be shifted by changing the working frequency and/or the cell configuration.

hydroxide. Application to the analysis of an acid mixture is shown in Fig. 23

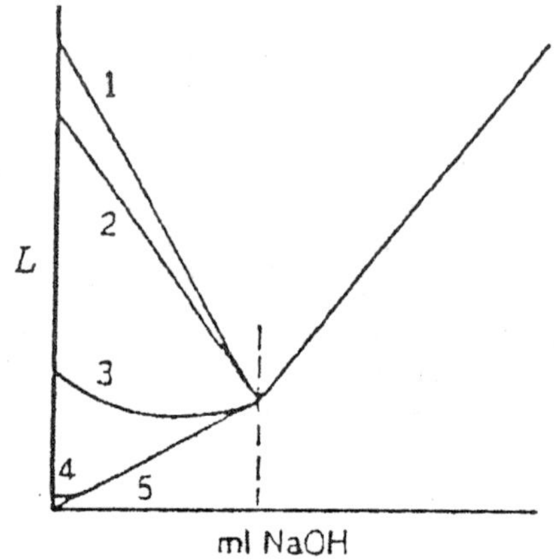

Fig.22: Conductometrci titration curves of various acids by sod. Hydroxide 1. hydrochloric acid, 2. dichloro acetic acid, 3. monochloroacetic acid, 4. acetic acid, and 5. boric acid

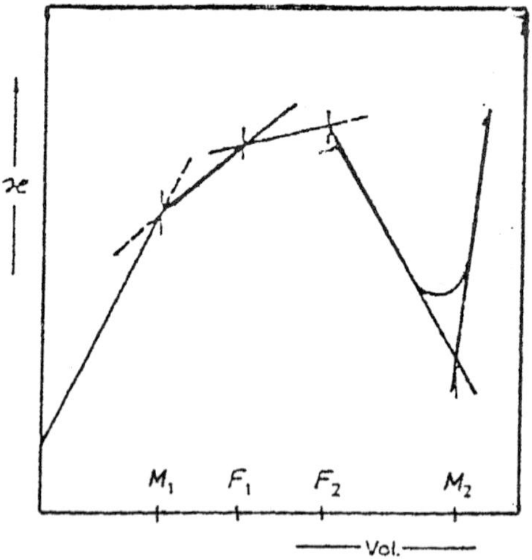

Fig.22: Differentiating titration of a mixture of fumaric acid (F) and maleic acid (M) in pyridine. The reagent for the titration is tetra-butylammonium hydroxide. Both steps in the dissociation of the weak acids can be observed.

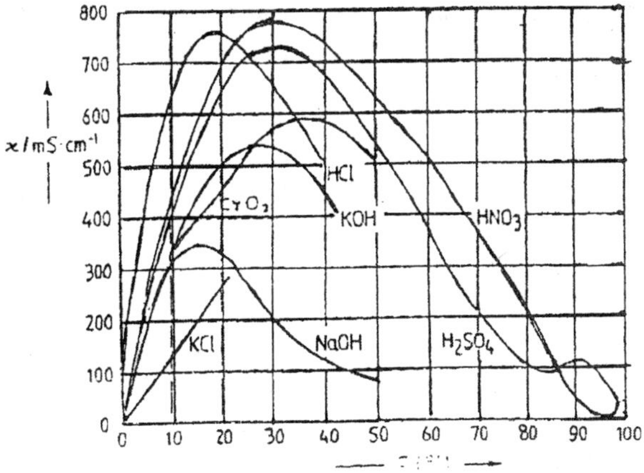

Fig.24: Conductivity plots (at 25°C) for strong electrolytes in most cases only the increasing part of the curves will be used. except in the case of sulphuric acid.

Table 4: Conductivity and Resistivity of Theoretically Pure Water

Temperature (°C)	**Conductivity (µS/cm)**	**Resistivity (MΩ- cm)**
0	0.01162	86.9
25	0.0550	18.18
50	0.1708	5.855
75	0.4010	2.494
100	0.7768	1.287

Conductivity detector is used in HPLC instrumentation. But, it is the most used detector for ion chromatography. A host of improvements have been made in cell design and detector circuitry, driven by the needs of this new analytical method. These include miniaturization of cell volume, improved electronic suppression and stabilization techniques, and better temperature control and

Table 5: Equivalent Conductances of some Electrolytes at 250C

Electrolyte	Concentration (Molarity)							
	0.0000	0.0005	0.001	0.005	0.01	0.02	0.05	0.10
Nacl	126.45	124.50	123.73	120.65	118.51	115.76	111.06	106.74
KCL	149.86	147.81	146.95	143.55	141.27	138.34	133.37	128.96
Li Cl	115.03	113.15	112.40	109.40	107.32	104.65	100.11	95.86
HCL	426.16	422.74	421.36	415.80	412.00	407.24	399.09	391.32
NH_4Cl	149.7	--	--	--	141.28	138.33	133.29	128.75
KBr	151.9	--	--	146.09	143.43	140.48	135.63	131.39
KI	150.3	--	--	144.37	142.18	139.45	134.97	131.11
NaI	126.94	125.36	124.25	121.25	199.24	116.70	112.79	108.78
NaO_2CCH_3	91.0	89.2	88.5	85.72	83.76	81.24	76.92	72.80
$NaO_2CCH_2CH_3$	85.92	84.24	83.54	80.90	79.05	76.63	--	--
$NaO_2C(CH_3)_2\ CH_3$	82.70	81.04	80.31	77.58	75.76	73.39	69.32	65.27
KNO_3	144.96	142.77	141.84	138.48	132.82	132.41	126.31	120.40
$KHCO_3$	118.00	116.10	115.34	112.24	110.08	107.22	--	--
$AgNO_3$	133.36	131.36	130.51	127.20	124.76	121.41	115.24	109.14
NaOH	248	246	245	240	237	233	227	221
H_2SO_4(a)	--	--	361	--	309	--	--	233
$1/2CaCl_2$	139.98	135.96	134.34	128.02	123.94	119.94	111.448	105.19
$1/2SrCl_2$	135.80	131.90	130.33	124.34	120.29	115.54	108.25	102.19
$1/2MgCl_2$	129.40	125.41	124.11	118.31	114.55	110.04	103.08	97.10
$1/2Ca(OH)_2$	258	--	--	233	226	214	--	--
$1/2NaSO_4$	129.9	125.74	124.15	117.15	112.44	106.78	97.75	89.98
$1/2NiSO_4$	--	118.7	113.1	93.2	82.7	72.3	59.2	50.8
$1/3LaCl_3$	145.9	139.6	137.0	127.5	121.8	115.3	106.2	99.1
$1/4KFe(CN)_6$	184	--	167.24	146.09	134.83	122.82	107.17	97.87

regulation. The principle of ion chromatography is shown in Fig. 25 while a typical ion chromatogram for analysis is given in Fig. 26. Table 6 shows compounds amenable to ion chromatographic analysis.

Amongst industrial applications, sulphuric acid presents an interesting case. In contact process sulpuric acid industry, the range of interest is from 95.5 to 99.0% which means that the descending part of conductivity curve following the second maximum is used.

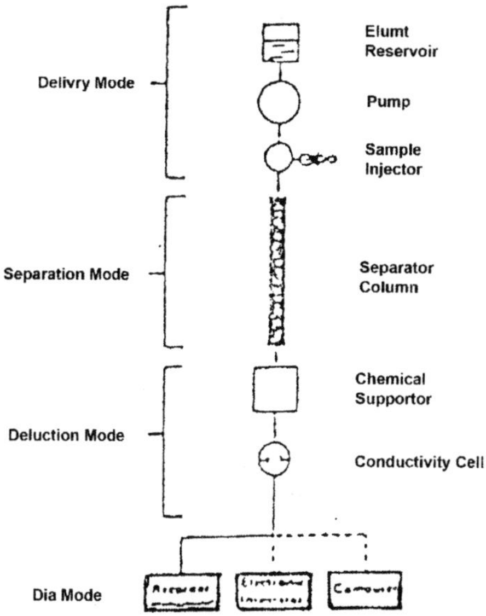

Fig. 25: A typical ion chromatogrph

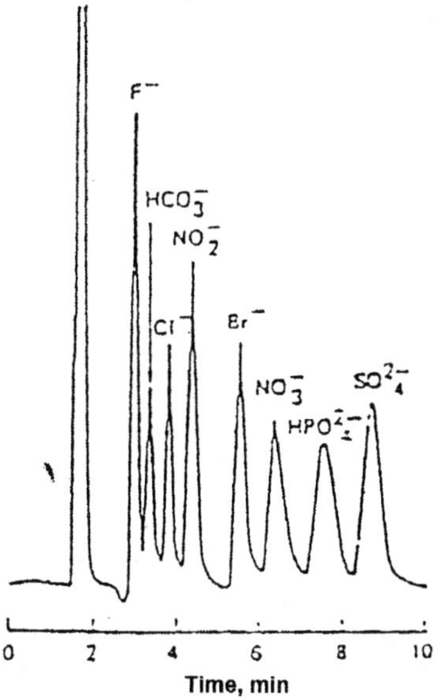

Fig. 26: A typical ion chromatogram for anaion analysis

Table 6: Some Compounds Amenable in Ion Chromatographic Analysis

Major Classes of Compounds	Examples	Primary Detectors
Inorganics	Sulfate, sulrite, thiosutrate, suride, hatices, nitrate, nitrite,borate, phosphate, hypophosphite, pyrophosphate, tripolysulfate, trimetaphosphate, selenate, selenite, arsenate, arsenite, chlorite, perchlorate, chlorate, hypochlorite, carbonate, cyanide	**Conductivity Amperometry**
Metals	Alkalis, alkaline earths, gold (I and II), platinum, silver, palladium, iron (II and III), copper, nickel, tin, lead, cobalt, manganese, cadmium, chromium, aluminium	**Conductivity Colorimetry**
Organics	Organic acids, amines, amino acids, carbohydrates, alcohol, saccharin, sugars, surfactants (anionic or cationic)	**Conductivity Amperometry Fluorescence**

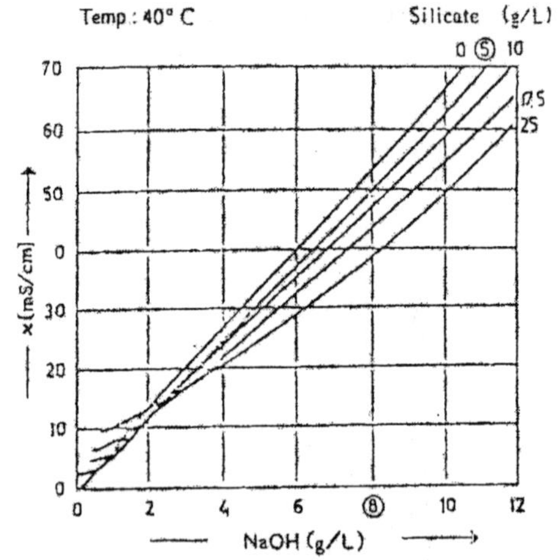

Fig.27: Conductivity plot of a system with two dissolved electrolytic components. The best way to bleach raw cotton is with hydrogen peroxide, which makes no contribution to the conductivity of the bleach liquor. To stabilize the bleaching baths caustic soda (NaOH) and silicate (water-glass) have to be added. The main contribution to the conductivity is form NaOH. Therefore, replenishment of NaOH is based on conductivity measurements.

Interestingly, the conductivity of concentrated sulphuric acid in low (-10mS/ cm) and such solutions behave equally well as an electrolyte and as a hydrogen-bonded liquid with "nearly organic" properties. The conductivity cell for such applications must be careful designed, with a strong preference for contactless inductive cells.

Another typical application is the concentration monitoring of hydrogen peroxide bleach liquor for cotton fabrics. The process is run at higher pH values where the peroxide is liable to deteriorate. The liquor therefore has to be stabilized by addition of water-glass (sodium tetrasilicate), which itself is an electrolyte. Fig. 27 shows the behaviour of such a multi-component system.

The use of conductivity of water as a quality parameter and in water treatment is summarized in Table 7.

Table 7: Conductivity of water as quality parameter and in water treatment

Parameter/ Process	Procedure
Total dissolved salts of surface water	The conductivity (S/cm) leads to the concentratic c = $6.4.10^5 \cdot k$ (mg./L) Bottger equation
Chlorinity of sea water	Ther chlorinity Cl can be estimated out of salinity S (Both in ppt) with direct reading conductivity instruments : Cl= (S - 0.03) / 1.385
Purity of stream condensate using water cooled condensers	Sampling through a cartridge of an ion-exchanger in the H^{+-} form, converting all cations into H^+ - ions (increased sensitivity)
Effluent monitoring of Ion-exchanges for water-desalinitation	a) Continuous effluent monitoring indicates the break-through. b) rinsing of the regenerated exchangers by conductivity control
Rinsing water control	Fresh-water replenishment of rinsing baths in plating shops with "water savers" (Closed control loop conductivity measurement)

15

CENTRIFUGE

Centrifuges are designed to accelerate the sedimentation process by utilizing centrifugal force. Various types of centrifuges are used in the clinical laboratory for separating suspended particles from a liquid in which the particles are not soluble. Liquids of differing specific gravity may also be separated on a centrifuge. There are three types of centrifuges: the horizontal rotor, the fixed-angle rotor, and the ultracentrifuge. Variations of the first two include bench-top and floor-standing units, high-speed units, refrigerated units. Special-purpose equipment include microhematocrit, cell washer, cytospin, and continuous-flow systems.

In the clinical laboratory, the centrifuge functions as a filtration or packing device. The development of large-batch centrifuges and continuous-flow systems that can sediment a precipitate from a large volume of solution in a short time has tended to replace the tedious process of filtration in most clinical and research laboratories. Coupled with refrigeration, this has reduced sample lability to a minimum.

General applications include the separation of serum or plasma from red blood cells, separation of precipitated solids from the liquid phase of a mixture, or separation of liquids of varying density. Special purpose units include applications such as:

quantitative blood cells packing for measuring hematocrit, automatic cell washing, and component preparation for blood banking. Ultracentrifuges employ very high speed and force to achieve difficult and precise quantitative separations of ultra small particles or macromolecules.

The horizontal rotor centrifuge shields or cups are in a vertical position when the centrifuge is at rest and assume a horizontal position when it is operating. The horizontal rotor unit will operate at speeds up to about 3000 rpm. Speeds higher than this can be attained but are not generally practical because of the excess heat developed by air friction. Depending upon the radius of the rotor, the units attain forces of approximately 1650 g.

The fixed-angle rotor centrifuge shields or cups are positional rigidly at a fixed angle, generally 25° or 50°, to the shaft around which they rotate. Angle rotor units may attain much higher speeds. This is due to the special construction of the rotor, which exhibits very low friction with air. The cups are enclosed by a metal case that reduces wind resistance, minimizing the increase of sample temperature. They can reach speeds of about 7000 rpm and can exhibits forces > 9000 g.

In the horizontal rotor configuration, the particles being sediment must travel the entire length of the column of liquid to reach the bottom of the tube. As the containers fall from the horizontal to vertical position when the centrifuge stops, a remixing of the sediments and the solution can occur. In the fixed angle rotor centrifuge, this is not the case. With the shields and cups at a fixed angle, the particles have a shorter distance to travel, i.e. across the column of liquid to the side of the container. These particles from clusters and move to the bottom of the container very rapidly. The fixed-angle rotor centrifuge is a more efficient means of sedimentation.

High-speed micro centrifuges incorporate either fixed angle or horizontal rotors of small radius. With sample volumes of upto

2 ml., they are capable of speeds to 15000 rpm and forces up to 15000xg. Refrigerated centrifuges are available in both bench-type and floor model. They have internal refrigeration systems capable of maintaining temperatures ranging from - 15°C to 25°C during centrifugation. They may incorporate either fixed-angle or horizontal rotors. Refrigeration permits separation at higher speeds by protecting samples from heat generated during centrifugation.

Centrifuges capable of producing speeds up to 1,00,000 rpm with relative centrifugal force (RCF) values of 6,00,000xg, are referred to as ultracentrifuges. Both fixed-angle and horizontal rotors are used in them. In addition, some instruments have vertical rotor in which the axis of the tubes is fixed parallel to the rotor's axis of rotation. Even with the high forces produced, several hours or even days are required to obtain complex separations under controlled temperatures. The general centrifugation techniques utilizing the ultracentrifuge include differential, rate zonal, and isospylenic separations. Differential centrifugation separates particles from a mixture by sedimenting those of larger mass to the bottom, leaving a portion of the small particles in the supernatant. The rate zonal technique separates particle based on differences in sedimentation rate in a density gradient, such as sucrose. The isopylenic technique separates particles based on difference in density (composition) in a density gradient, such as caesium chloride. The large centrifuge is significantly more complex than general laboratory centrifuges.

One variety off the ultracentrifuge used in clinical laboratories, is the Airfuge (Beckman) which is a miniature ultracentrifuge. It uses a small turbine rotor driven by air pressure. It is capable of speed up to 95000 rpm and forces up to 1,78,000xg. The rotor spins nearly friction-free on a cushion of air, and temperature can be controlled by the temperature of the drive air. A variety of rotors are available. General applications include receptor assays, protein fractionation, and drug-binding assays.

Perhaps the most common clinical laboratory application is the classification of lipemic sera.

Selection of a centrifuge:

This is based on the number and volume of samples to be separated during a run and at what RCF? Other considerations include physical size, rotor versatility, timing and refrigeration needs, frequency of use, and maintenance requirements.

Components:

The parts of a common centrifuge include the chamber which encloses the internal parts, a cover with latch, the centrifugal rotor with shields or cups, and the motor driven assembly. Most centrifuges will include a power switch, a braking device, speed control, a timer, and possibly, a tachometer.

Centrifuge motors are either series-wound dc motors that turn faster as voltage is increased or ac motors in which speed adjustment is achieved through stepwise reduction of the number of poles in the magnetic field. Both types are higher speed motors that generally employ direct-drive systems to the rotor through the motor shaft.

Electrical contact to the commutator in nearly all centrifuge motors is provided by graphite brushes, which gradually wear down as they press against the commutator turning at high speed. If the graphite is allowed to completely wear away, the retainer spring of the brush will make contact with the smooth surface of the commutator and will cut grooves or scratches in its surface. A rough commutator surface will cause excessively fast wear of new brushes. The graphite that is worm away may deposit around the contacts, causing arcing and burning, both of which decrease the efficiency of the motor and may damage it or, in extreme cases, may even start a fire in the motor. The shaft of the motor turns through sleeve bearings located at the top and bottom of the rotor.

Most units contain sealed bearings that are permanently lubricated, whereas others require periodic oil or grease. Many centrifuges contain an internal imbalance switch that turns the unit off before vibrations from local imbalance can damage bearings on the drive shaft.

The speed of the centrifuge is controlled by a potentiometer, which raises and lowers the voltage supplied to the motor. The calibrations furnished on the speed control of a centrifuge are often only relative voltage increments and can never be taken as accurate indicators of speed. Because speed is dependent upon voltage in most centrifuges, as resistance is increased speed is lost. Air resistance and turbulence, brush friction, and electrical inefficiency of the centrifuge itself are sources of resistance. These resistances can cause a centrifuge to operate at differing speeds on the same speed-control rating. Different accessories, loads, and varying states of repair will also result in the same speed control problems. Calibration and periodic recalibration of centrifuge speed is extremely important.

Operating a centrifuge with the lid raised is dangerous and must be discouraged. In addition to being hazardous and reducing the centrifuge's speed through increased air resistance, it also causes the revolving parts of the centrifuge to vibrate excessively. Vibrations cause extensive wear on the centrifuge and a remixing of the sediment particles.

Tachometers are provided on many centrifuges to indicate the speed in rpm. On mechanical tachometers, a flexible shaft or cable attached to the motor spindle turns inside a flexible housing to which the motor movement is attached at the end. As the cable turns, it causes the needle to move up-scale. Modern centrifuges use electric tachometers in which a magnet rotates around a coil, producing a current that may be measured of a tachometer is not attached to the centrifuge, a stroboscope or an electronic meter can be used to determine the actual rpm of each centrifuge setting. For any given setting, the speed of the centrifuge will very with the specimen load. The rpm determined for each centrifuge setting should be recorded and attached to the centrifuge for easy reference.

The value of rpm is only one factor involved in determining centrifugal force. The true efficiency of a particular centrifuge is expressed in relative centrifugal force, some number times gravity. The relative centrifugal force is calculated from the experimentally determined rpm and the radius of the rotor plus carrier.

The term rpm, when applied to a centrifuge, does not give any indication of the force applied to samples in that centrifuge. All comparisons made between centrifuges should be in relative centrifugal force. When an RCF (relative centrifugal force) value specified in a procedure cannot be obtained on a particular centrifuge, it is possible to adjust the length of time in which samples are centrifuged to achieve equivalent centrifugal force. Time required can be calculated as follows :

$$T = \frac{T_S \times RCF_S}{RCE}$$

Where :

T = run time needed

T_s = run time specified in a procedure

RCF = RCF obtainable

RCF_s = RCF specified in a procedure

Relative centrifugal force (RCF): A method of comparing the forces generated by various centrifuges, considering the speed of rotation and the radius from the centre of rotation. Relative centrifugal force is calculated according to the formula,

$$RCF = 1.12\ r\ (rpm / 1000)^2$$

A timer device is commonly employed in many centrifuges. Some are spring-driven clock mechanisms that turn the unit off after a present time cycle. Others are electronic timers that perform the same function. Many units have switches that allow units to be operated continuously without using the timer device.

Braking devices are incorporated to provide rapid deceleration of the unit. Two general types of brake mechanisms are found on centrifuges. One type is mechanical and functions by physically applying pressure to the rotor at some point when a lever is pressed. The other type, found on most units, is electrical in nature and functions by reversing the polarity of the current to the motor.

BLOCK SCHEMATIC OF A TYPICAL

REFRIGERATED CENTRIFUGE

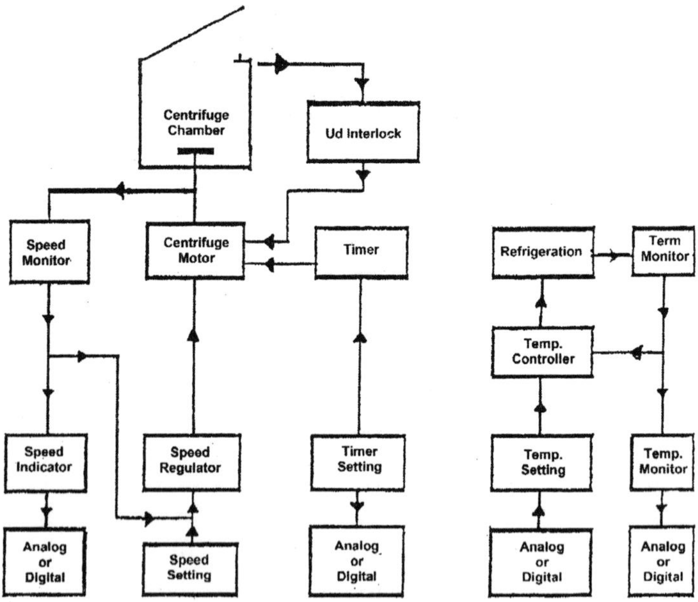

Centrifuges: General Operation and Maintenance

Daily operation along with periodic function verification and proper preventive maintenance are vital to the efficiency and longevity of the centrifuge. A regular schedule for checks must be drawn and followed to ensure proper operation of the equipment.

Daily operation:

Daily operation should include observation and inspection of the following

1. The centrifuge should not be on the same circuit as sensitive electronic measuring devices, such as spectrophotometers, because it generates electronic noise and has a high current drain when started up. The unit should not be near combustible fluids as ignition may occur from sparking motor brushes.
2. Check the cleanliness of the chamber, and immediately clean up all spills. Be aware of biohazardous materials (microbiological, radioactive, and chemical) that require specific decontamination procedures. Observe for gray or black dust build-up within the chamber; this can be a sign of sandblasting of the rotor chamber caused by glass particles and must be cleaned up promptly. Refrigerated units will require periodic defrosting.
3. Always balance the load of the centrifuge before operating; use the correct tube sizes and types for the particular centrifuge. The load must be balanced both by equal mass and by centre of gravity across the centre of rotation. Do not run the centrifuge with buckets, carriers or shields missing from the unit.
4. Always make sure that the cover is closed while the unit is operating. This will help prevent the dangerous aerosolization of biohazardous and scattering of physically dangerous material into the environment. Centrifuge only sealed or Stoppered tubes if possible.
5. Observe for unusual noises or vibrations during operation. Do not operate the unit in excess of the maximum speed recommended by the manufacturer for the rotor in use.

Vibrations occur naturally during acceleration and deceleration at low speeds. This is the critical speed range of the rotor and is generally in the range 500 to 1000 rpm. Avoid prolonged operation within this range.

6. Never open the chamber until the rotor has come to a complete stop.

Preventive maintenance:

Preventive maintenance should be performed on the same time schedule as function verification procedures. It should include the following:

1. ***Lubrication***: Depending upon the type of centrifuge, bearings on the upper and lower end of the motor shaft may be permanently lubricated or sealed. If they are not sealed, the manufacturer's instructions must be followed for lubrication. Bearing wear may be checked at this time by determining the amount of side play in the shaft.
2. ***Motor components:*** Brushes should be removed and checked for wear. Replacement is recommended if they are worn to more than one-half their original length. When reinserting used brushes, replace them in the same orientation and be certain that spring tension is adequate to maintain good contact with the commutator. New brushes should be broken in by accelerating the unloaded unit slowly to mid-speed and by allowing it to operate this way for a period of time. The condition of the commutator should be examined. To avoid electrical arcing, the commutator and brush holders must be free of dirt, oil and dust. severe arcing of new brushes can be a sign of a bad commutator. If the commutator is scratched or scored, it will have to be removed and machined smooth with a lathe or replaced. On refrigerated units, the manufacturer's instruction manual should be consulted for maintenance procedures on the refrigeration system.

3. ***Electrical integrity:*** Both grounding resistance and current leakage should be checked periodically on each centrifuge. The fuse should be checked for proper rating; if the unit has a circuit-beaker, it should be checked for proper operation. In addition, the line cord, plug, lamps, and wiring should be examined for defects.
4. ***Mechanical integrity:*** If the unit is equipped with a safety interlock, this device should be checked for proper working order. Gaskets, latches, hinges, and control knobs should be examined to determine that all are functioning and are in good condition. The rotor and shields or carriers should be examined for any signs of mechanical stress (cracks, corrosion) and for cleanliness and balance.

Function verification:

The function verification procedures should be appropriate for the application of the centrifuge. It is generally recommended that such procedures be performed at 1 to 3 month intervals, with more frequent checks for the units with critical applications. Correction factors for speed, timing, or temperature should be posted on the unit.

Tolerance limits for function checks should be established. These will again depend on the applications. Information for corrective action should the tolerance limits be exceeded, must be included. Function verification procedures should include the following:

1. ***rpm calibration:*** One of the best ways to check the function of a centrifuge is to check its speed. Depending upon how the unit is equipped, both the speed control and built- in tachometer should be checked with an external device, e.g. a stroboscope or a mechanical or electronic tachometer of good accuracy. Several speeds used regularly on the unit should be checked. Values obtained with the external measuring device should agree within 5 % of those from a

built in tachometer. Centrifuges that cannot be checked without opening the chamber lid should be tested by factory-trained personnel only.

Time: the timer should be set for common timing intervals and these intervals should be checked against an accurate stopwatch or electronic timer. The timing interval includes

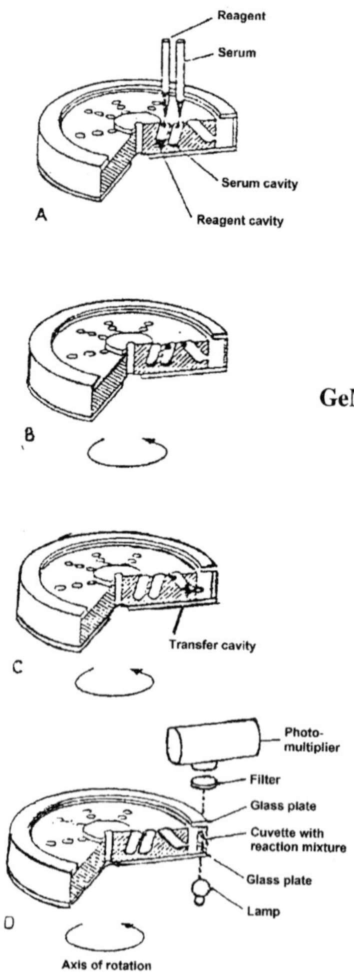

Centrifuge Analyzer for Clinical Analysis

Use of centrifugal force to add, transfer and mix reagent and sample.

Samples processed in parallel cavities in a modified centrifuge head with an optical cuvette for each sample, along its wall.

High volume analysis possible (up to 420 samples per hour)

Microvolumes of reagent used : low cost per sample

GeMSAEC fast analyzer transfer disk

(A) Sample and reagent are measured in to chambers where they remain separate and unmixed at rest and during rotation at low speed.

(B) As speed is increased, both liquids begin to move radially into outer chamber of transfer disk.

(C) Liquids flow rapidly out of transfer disk and into cuvettes in cuvette rotor.

(D) The reactant solutions are held against the outer walls of the cuvette and air bubbles are displaced from the mixtures by centrifugal displacement.

Optical measurements may now begin.

the period of acceleration and spin, but not brake or stopping time. General laboratory centrifuges should be accurate to 10 % of the total timed interval.

Temperature: The thermometer on refrigerated units should be checked against a certified thermometer, and a correction factor should be derived if necessary.

16

BALANCE

Matter: The earth and its envelope is made up of matter. It is characterized by gravitational properties like weight.

Mass and density: All substances have mass. For any given volume that mass remains constant and can be defined as "quantity of matter in a body" independent of gravitational force.

Weight: A body has weight because it is pulled toward the center of the earth by the force of gravity and the amount of that body weighs is a measure of that pull.

$F = ma$, but here a = g (Acceleration due to gravitational force of the earth = 32.2 ft/sec^2) in the latitude of 45° i.e. at sea level. Weight is a vector quantity has both magnitude as well as direction. The "poundal" is that force which produces an acceleration of one foot per second each second in a mass of one pond.

Center of gravity: The gravitational force exerts its influence on all particles of a body. Thus, in the case of a bar of metal, which is in a plane of horizontal, every particle being acted upon by a similar and parallel active force. If we support the bar so that there is an equal distribution of mass on either side of the center of support the bar will remain horizontal. The slightest disturbance of the bar will cause rotation about the center of suspension, the bar ultimately coming to rest with the center of its mass bellow the center of suspension, giving a state of stable equilibrium.

When a body is supported at its center of mass in remains in an inert position, i.e. one of neutral equilibrium.

Moment of a force = Force X arm

Conditions to be satisfied in beam scale construction:

1. The arms of the unloaded beam must have equal moments about the fulcrum.
2. The parts suspended from the end knife-edges must be of equal weight.
3. The knife-edges must be equidistant from, and parallel to, the fulcrum knife-edge.
4. The center of gravity of the unloaded assembly should be bellow and on the perpendicular through, the fulcrum knife-edge.
5. The smaller the distance between the center of gravity and the fulcrum knife-edge, the greater the sensitivity, subject always to maintenance of stability.
6. The longer the arms the greater the sensitivity.
7. Lighter the beam less the inertia factor, normally opposing the quick response.
8. The fulcrum knife-edge must be slightly below the line joining the end knife-edges.
9. Friction between knife-edges and bearings should be reduced to a minimum.

STEELYARDS:

Steelyard is an unequal arm balance. When no load is suspended from the load hook *A* or the blade *BD*, the center of gravity of the whole may be assumed to be at *G*. If we use *W* to denote the weight of the unloaded steel yard, then, in order to nullify the moment (*W*

X *GF*) acting in a counter-clockwise direction, we must suspend at *B*, a weight *C* of such value that (*C* X *BF*) = (*W* X *GF*), in which event the center of gravity of the system is now in the vertical through *F*. The weight *C* is our movable and position *B* is the zero graduation in our weight-registering system.

If we suspend a load *L* from *A*, we will need to move *C* out ward from *F* until equilibrium is restored. Let us assumed that this is achieved when *C* is at position *D*.

The equation of moment is now:

$$(L \times AF) + (G \times GF) = (C \times BF) + (C \times BD).$$

But, $W \times GF = C \times BF$

Therefore, $L \times AF = C \times BD$

or, $L = (C \times BD) / AF$

C and *AF* are constants, therefore *BD* is directly proportional to the load *L*. From this it will be seen that if we divide *BD* in to equal intervals of distance then each will represent an identical weight value.

Requirements of a precision balance:

Truth:

The beam is horizontal i.e. in equipoise, both when unloaded and when equal masses are freely suspended from the terminal knife-edges.

Stability:

This requirement is satisfied when the beam, if disturbed from the equilibrium position tends to return the original position of rest.

Sensitivity:

This requirement is satisfied when a small difference in load suspended from the terminal knife-edges causes an appreciable movement of the beam from horizontal.

Truth:

If the beam is horizontal i.e. in equipoise, both when unloaded and when equal masses are freely suspended from the terminal knife-edges of the beam. This can be assured by the following equalities:

(a) The moments of the weights of the two arms of the beam about the fulcrum, measures from their respective centers of gravity.

(b) The weights of the two scale-pans with their suspension fittings.

(c) The moment arms of the terminal knife-edges about the fulcrum knife-edge.

In the event of condition (a) not being satisfied, the beam will not maintain equivocation when unloaded.

If (b) is not satisfied the same result would be obtained. If possible for neither (a) nor (b) to be satisfied and the unloaded beam to remain horizontal, due to moment of beam arms and the suspended parts exactly canceling each other. If however, the suspended parts are reversed the two errors become combined.

If condition (c) is not satisfied, inequality of the moment arms of the terminal knife-edges will be apparent when known equal masses are suspended from those knife-edges.

Stability: If the beam is disturbed from the equilibrium position should tend to return its original position of rest. To ensure this, the contact line of the fulcrum knife-edge must be above the center of gravity of the beam.

If the center of gravity coincides with the fulcrum, the bean will be in a condition of neutral equilibrium and will remain in any position in which it is placed.If the center of gravity of the beam, when horizontal, is immediately above the fulcrum, the beam will be unstable and will accelerate away from the horizontal if disturbed. In this condition attainment of equipoise is difficult and its maintenance is impossible in the presence of slightest disturbance.

Fulcrum is in the same plane as the terminal knife-edges.

Fulcrum is bellow the line joining the terminal knife-edges.

Fulcrum is above the line joining the terminal knife-edges.

Sensitivity: This requirement is satisfied when a small differenc in loades suspended from the terminal knife-edges causes an appreciable movement of the beam from horizontal.

(a) The longer the arm (L) of the beam greater the sensitivity.

(b) The less the weight (W) of the beam the greater the sensitivity.

(c) The nearer the center of gravity of the beam to the fulcrum, i.e. the smaller the distance (d) , the greater the sensitivity.

$$\text{Tan } \alpha = \frac{L}{W \times d}$$

17

SINGLE PAN BALANCE

A. PRINCIPLE:

A single pan balance is an unequal arm balance in which weights are lifted instead of being added. When we weigh on a two pan balance, we place counter weights and measure in an equal arms arrangement. When we place some mass on the sample cell/pan of a single or monopan balance, a deflection is produced which is measured with reference to a line/mark upon another scale or screen which is the image of the projection scale mounted on the damping side of the beam.

B. CONSTRUCTION:

A beam of light from a lamp passes through a field lens, condensed on a projection scale and then the image of the scale is focused on the screen by a projection lens system in between the scale and the screen. There may be reflector to rotate the image at right angle towards the screen. The projection scale is a 0 – 100 division scale of some special unit, e.g. 1 division representative 10 mg or 1 mg, as per specification. Without any mass on to the sample pan, zero of the image scale should coincide with the reference line on the screen.

When there is a small deflection due to the unknown mass, its magnitude can be seen on the screen upto 100 mg. when the unknown sample weight is more than 100 mg, nothing is observed on the screen. Manipulation knobs are then used to lift vertical and horizontal ring weights by weight lifters to bring the scale on the screen, and the weights can be seen on the manipulation circular scales. Most balances have capacity upto 99.999 g – 100 g and a sensitivity of 0.001 g. The stirrup upon which the horizontal and vertical weights are suspended is also called the weight carriage.

C. FIGURES OF MERIT:

Damping screw and Gravity screw: The requirements like 'truth' (or accuracy) 'stability' and 'sensitivity' of a balance are controlled by adjustment of "G" centre of gravity by the damping screw and gravity screw. The knife edges are made from finely polished agate. Levelling screws are provided to level the balance for free movement and the levelling is checked by the spirit level provided onboard.

D. CALIBRATION OF BALANCE:

The balance is calibrated with the help of properly preserved standard weights. A series of weights covering the entire weighing range (capacity) of the balance.

E. MAINTENANCE AND CARE OF THE BALANCE :

Handling of a single pan balance requires greater care, skill and patience as the balance consists of several precision optical and mechanical components. The following defects/malfunctioning may occur, mainly due to bad handling or carelessness:

1. ***Projection lamp may not be illuminated***: electrical connections may be checked; lamp life may be over
2. ***image of the graticule not on the screen***:
    i) Beam may not be sitting in the proper place

ii) Image is not focused

iii) Stirrup and weights may be disturbed

iv) Reflecting prism on mirror may be disturbed

3. ***The projection scale does not move freely***:

i) Ring riders may have slipped from the hanger

ii) Balance may not be properly leveled

iii) Stirrup may be disturbed / displaced

4. ***Main scale zero does not coincide with reference line***:

i) Adjust using side adjustment screw but do not touch the gravity screws

ii) Level the instrument properly

5. ***Image is not clear***: Clean the optical system: mirror, plane parallel plate, etc. with acetone. The graticule should be cleaned carefully with soft brush

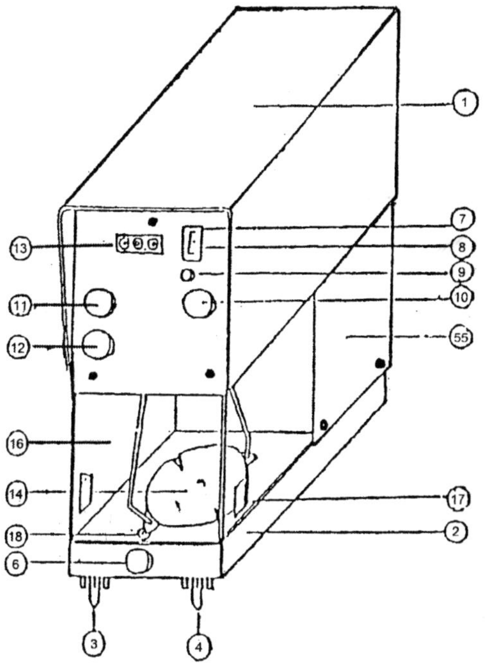

FIGURE FRONT VIEW OF THE BALANCE

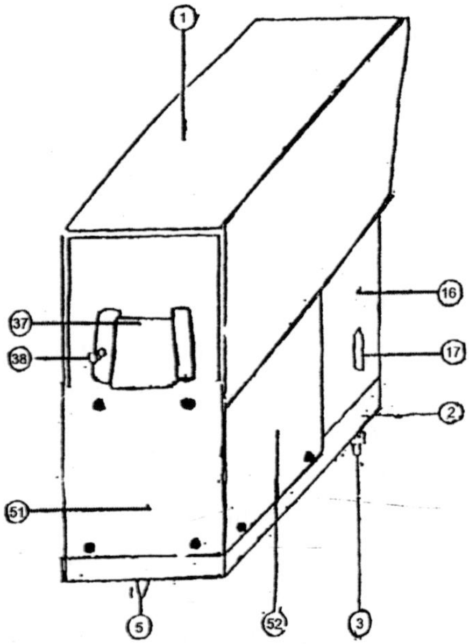

FIGURE BACK VIEW OF SINGLE PAN BALANCE

1. Top cover of balance
2. Base of the balance
3. Left side leg screw
4. Right side leg screw
5. Back leg pin
6. Operation knob

   G - R Rest position of operating knob

   G - O Checking position of operation knob

   G - W weighing position of operating knob
7. Ground glass screen with vernler scale
8. Vernler scale graduation
9. Vernler scale operating knob
10. First declinal place manipulation knob
11. Unit gramme place manipulation knob

12. Tenth gramme place manipulation knob
13. Weight indicator tabular scale
14. Stainless steel pan
15. Pan rest
16. Glass side doors
17. Glass door Handles
18. Spirit level
19. Weight Carriage
20. Hanger rod for ring riders
21. Horizontal ring riders (Weights)
22. Vertical ring riders, unit gramme place
23. Vertical ring riders, first decinal gramme place
24. Lifters for horizontal weights
25. Lifters for vertical ring riders
26. Beam with damping plate
27. Dampling plate
28. Graduated projection scale
29. Projection scale image
30. Side adjustment screws
31. Gravity scerws
32. Central knife-edge of beam
33. Stirrup sideknife-edge of beam
34. Rest support for beam, damping end
35. Rest support for beam, stirrup end
36. Leg rcats
37. Rear panel housing for projection lamp
38. Rear housing knob
39. Projection lamp
40. Projection lamp holder
41. Projection bulb carriage

42. Scerw for projection lamp carriage
43. Connecting terminal to the projection lamp
44. Left side total reflecting prism
45. Right side total reflecting prism
46. Right side prism stand
47. Stirrup
48. Hanger for pan
49. Transformer
50. Connecting terminals to transformer output
51. Connecting terminals to transformer Input
52. Connecting terminals to main source output
53. Front panel
54. Rear Housing of base
55. Rear housing side paltes
56. Operating knob housing benenth the base
57. Magnifier
58. Adjustment screw of the right and side prism stand
59. Dampling cup
60. Agate base for central knife -edge.

18

PROJECTORS

Projector is an instrument which projects recorded photographic image or any matter upon a slide. These are also used for inspection of small engineering components with a profile or scale on the screen, known as profile projector.

For a good projector portrait lenses are used as projection lens for 8mm, 16mm and 35mm films, which must have very high standard of reproduction capacity. A field flattener is some time added to reduce the petzval curve and therefore the optical system plays an important role.

A small change in optical axis can damage the quality of the image. In most of the slide projectors quartz–iodine tungsten lamps are used as the source, which can emit infrared with visible radiation and therefore, heat filters are kept in between lamp and optical system. Small fan is also fixed inside the slide projector near the lamp to save the life of the lamp from excess heat.

The focal length of the condenser is matched with the film size and lens aperture. For sufficient illumination at the frame the adjustment of the light source is essential.

Modern slide projectors have the facilities to bring the slide in front of projection lens and also to remove by automatic control switch; auto focus arrangements are also attached. These types of projectors may be connected with computers which can directly projects the matter on the screen.

Epidiascope:

Some time Epidiascopes are also used as projectors, but they are mainly useful for opaque objects, like books, etc., which can be directly protected on the screen. All these projectors require a precision optical system and Fresnel lens is an alternative to optical lens system.

Projection Lens:

Projection lenses have a great deal with camera lenses, but there are differences. Camera lenses are not very good for projecting an image, as projection lens requires longer focal length and narrow field angles. The relative apertures range from F/3.5 to F/1.5. The most widely used system for projecting transparencies is the Koehlar system. The source is assumed to be a disc of light source, which is Lambertian.

The diagram shows that two rays traced through an optical system. The 'a' ray starts at the center of the light source and is imaged to the projection system and the passes on to the projection screen. The 'b' ray passes through the center of the slide plane, expands to the projection lens, and is focused on the projection screen. From the optical invariant equation,

$$S \sin U_0 - D \sin U_2$$

The luminance on the screen is given by,

$$E = \pi B \sin^2 U_2$$

Where,

'B' is the luminance of the source (lumens / solid angle/ cm.)

The luminance can be written

$$E = \pi B\ (S/D)^2 \sin^2 U_0$$

The Equation shows that the luminance on the screen depends on the source luminance, the square of U_0 (referred to as the collection angle of the condenser), and the ratio of source diameter to the screen diameter.

He real situation is not possible as light sources are not exactly flat discs with Lambertian luminance, therefore rays are aberrated and the screen is not uniformly illuminated. The net result is that projection systems require uniform high –luminance source. Tungsten, carbon arc and high-pressure gas / mercury sources are today's choice.

Ground and opal glass can do a good job but it reduces the intensity. Some time light integrating bars are also used to collect all the rays like integrating sphere. The bar integrator is like a kapleidoscope.

The size of the independent source point is determined by NA of the condenser.

$$D = 1.22\ \lambda / U_0$$

Fresnel lens:

Fresnel lens was invented by French Physicist Augustin Jean Fresnel, who first used this design to build a glass house lens in 1822. The Fresnel lens is equivalent of a conventional optical lens; it is a thin flat special optical lens, which consists of a series of small narrow concentric grooves on the surface. Light weight plastic such as acrylic Polymethyl Methacrylate (PMMA), Polyvinyl chloride (PVC), Polycarbonate (PC) are used in order to reduce the thickness, weight and cost.

Each groove is at slightly different angle than the next and with the same in order to focus the light toward a central focal point. Every groove can be considered as an individual small lens. To bend parallel light waves, and focus the light. The lens actually eliminates some spherical aberration. Refractive index is about 1.492 and V- value is 57.4.

These lenses are light in weight and cost is about 40% less than glass lenses. The disadvantage of this type of lens is, it losses its stiffness above 80^0 C. Therefore it must be used where there is no excess heating.

A high groove density has a better quality projection image The Fresnel lens is a good solution for quality image and efficiency at a significantly lower cost. These lenses are corrected for spherical aberration.

Application of Fresnel lens: The application of Fresnel lens includes lighting lighthouse overhead projectors, Fresnel magnifier, TV projection, traffic sign, solar concentrator, collimator and LED.

Types of Fresnel lenses: Positive Fresnel lens, Negative Fresnel lens, Fresnel lens array, Clindrical Fresnel lens, Linear Fresnel lens, Fresnel reflection lens etc.

The ability accurately to project developed images is equally important as the initial recording on a photographic plate or film. Projectors are required for 8 mm, 16 mm and 35 mm motion pictures, 35 mm slide projectors, and For use with front or rear projection screens. Fig 1.

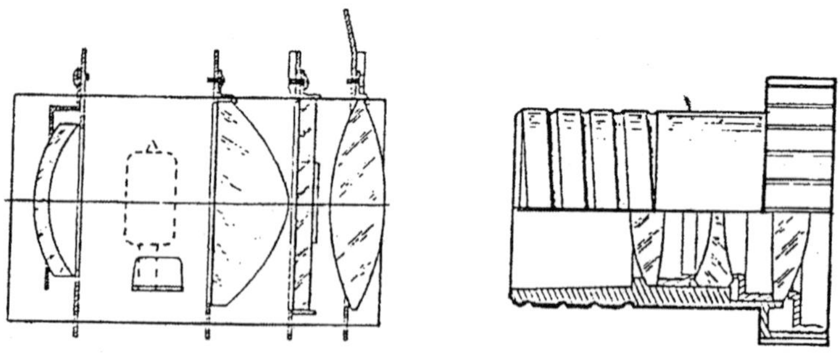

Fig.1: (a) Slide Projector Optical system including mirror quartz-iodine lamp flame-polished aspheric lens, heat filter, condenser lens and plastic mounted projection lens.

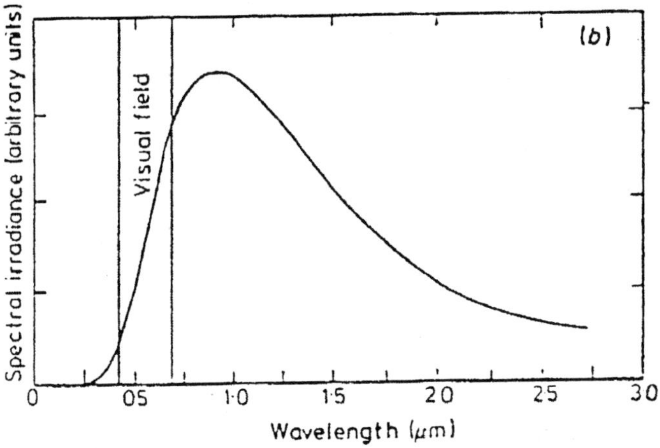

(b) Quartz iodine tungsten filament source spectral function.

Rear projectors are used for the inspection of small engineering components, in a workshop or view room, where the enlarged image is compared with a profile or scale on the font of the screen. Measurements on the screen image can be made with precision glass scales, as the divisions on the scale are magnified to correspond with the enlargement given by the lens in use. Fig.2

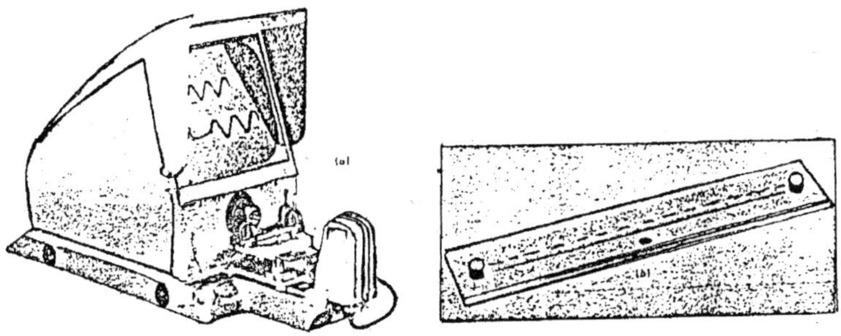

Fig.2: (a) The Projector for checking the dimensions of small components in the workshop, and detecting errors before they reach inspection department.

(b) The transport glass projector scale on the underside with magnification form 10X to 100X to suit projection lenses.

The portrait lenses designed by Joseph M.Petzval in 1840 has been modified for use as the most popular type of projection lens for 8 mm, 16 mm and 35 mm film. A high aperture lens at reasonable cost is possible with this design, as cine film projection does not require a wide angle of film. For 8 mm and 16 mm lenses a filed flattener is sometimes added to reduce the Petzvel curvature. Fig.3

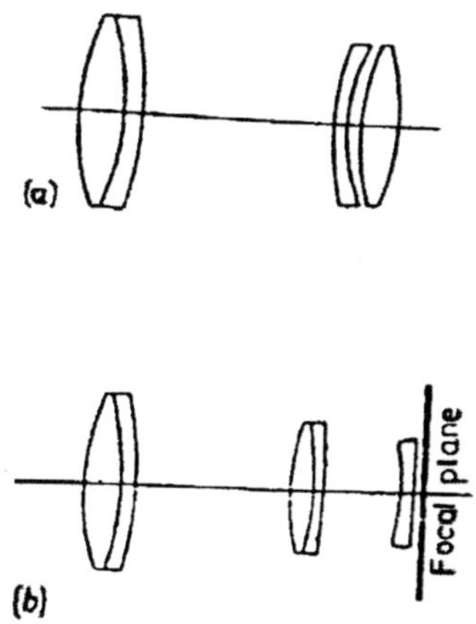

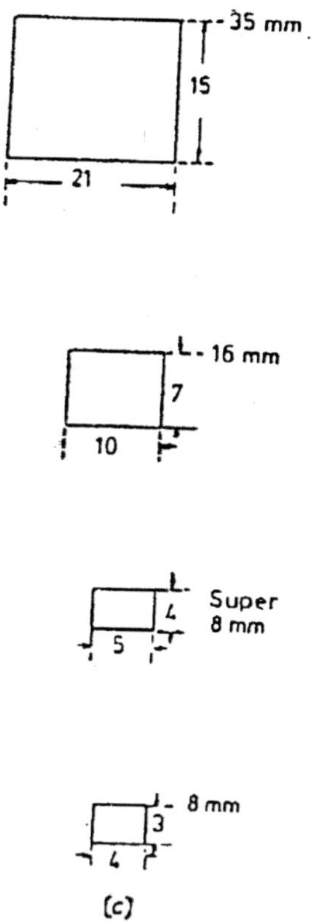

Fig.3: a. Petzvel lens as used in 35 mm motion-picture projection

b. Petzvel lenses with field flattener as used for 16 mm motion- picture projection.

c. Motion-picture projector aperture sizes, dimension in mm.

OVERHEAD PROJECTOR:

Overhead projection, a method of projecting transparencies has brought the overhead projector to very forefront of visual aid world. This instrument is very simple in concept and operation and helps people to communicate. For the lecture it brings new dimensions in teaching. A commercial overhead projector is a robust instrument of metal construction. A powerful tungsten halogen illumination source is used. Focusing is affected by rotating the large focusing knob conveniently located front of the instrument, which provides a smooth positive action and can be adjusted to individual requirements.

Access to projector interior can be obtained by releasing the slide catches and lift the top cover. This activate safety cutout double pole switch, which automatically cuts off electric supply.The Fresnel lens is easily is removable for cleaning and this also permits for both side of the glass plate. The tungsten halogen lamp operating through a built in transformer, bring all the advantages of low voltage illumination to over head projection and eliminate the need for a heat filter.

The Lamp: The lamp, the 'light source' is a halogen type made with a tungsten filament in a small quartz glass envelope filled with an iodine or bromide gas, and is specifically designed to run with a glass at a very high temperature. It has three advantages: a high white light output, it doses not blacken or change colour with age and it has an extra long life. This is because as tungsten vaporizes (it does not burn) instead of depositing on the glass, it combines with the halogen gas. This combination cannot be deposited on the high temperature glass and the tungsten is subsequently re-deposited back on the tungsten wire itself, thus extending of the filament life. The lamp should never be touched. The glass envelope runs at a very high temperature, and is not only dangerous but any oil or dirt at high temperature may dis-colour and will lower the light out put.

Lamp Type: Tungsten Halogen Philips 12260R or Equivalent. 240V, 600 Watts.

Thermostat Switch: A thermostat is provided in series with tungsten lamp. The thermostat is meant to cut-off the current or supply of lamp automatically when the projector becomes hot beyond the safe temperature limits. To reset the thermostat switch after it is cut-off, first allow the projector to become cool and press the reset button on the front panel. Listen for 'click' sound. The lamp will light again.

Light Control circuit: Light Control circuit may be incorporated to provide extra facility for desired intensity of light in any ambient condition. This light control unit helps to increase the lamp life by providing preheat condition as well as facility to operate lamp below the rated voltage. In this circuit, voltage across the lamp is controlled by the controlling conduction angle to the gate of triac. When the triac fires, the lamp get full voltage available at that phase angle. For the remaining period of that half cycle lamp will not get any voltage. Same thing repeats for other half cycle, if triac conducts for shorter period of phase angle lamp gets lesser average power and if triac conducts for longer period of phase angle, lamp gets more average power.

OVERHEAD PROJECTORS:

Overhead projectors use a moulded plastic Freznel condenser system. (J.D. Frezenl, 1788-1827). The Freznel lens is the equivalent of a conventional lens reproduced as series of rings impressed on the surface of an acrylic polymer moulding. Spherical, elliptical or parabolic surface can by produced with varying degrees of correction to suit the optical system. Fig.4.

Freznel lenses are light in weight and cost about 40% less than the glass lens equivalent in production quantities. A disadvantage is that this type of condenser lens will lose stiffness above 85°C so it can only be used where there is no excessive heating and the only important use is in overhead projectors.

A commercial overhead projector is shown in Fig. 5. It is a robust instrument of all metal construction, designed for rugged, hard-working use. The availability of projectors with a powerful

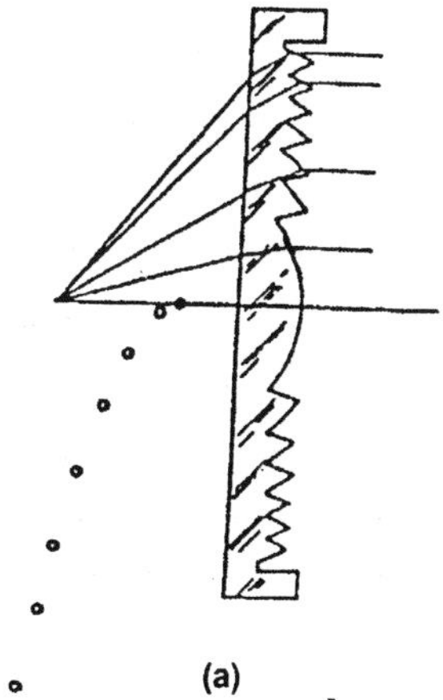

(a)

Fig. a: **Freznel lens consists of a central spherical or spherical form with circular zones surrounding the central lens, all having the same focal length and almost the same thickness. The center of curvature of the circular zones (marked as small circulars) do not lie on the optical axis. The radii of curvature increase with distance form the center as in an aspheric lens. The lens will give parallel rays of light, but dark annular spaces are formed by the dead areas between the circular zones.**

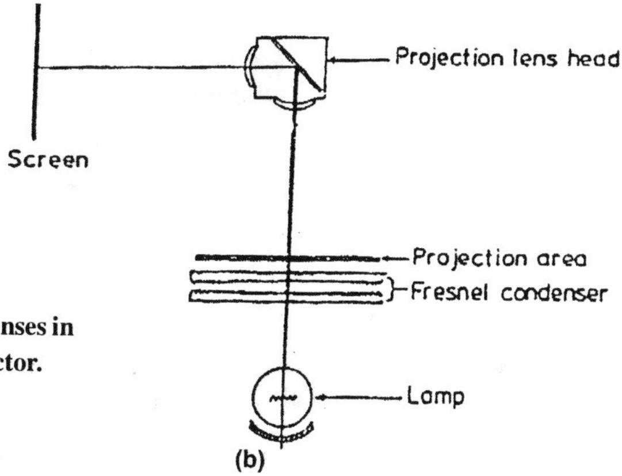

(b)

b. Use of Freznel lenses in overhead projector.

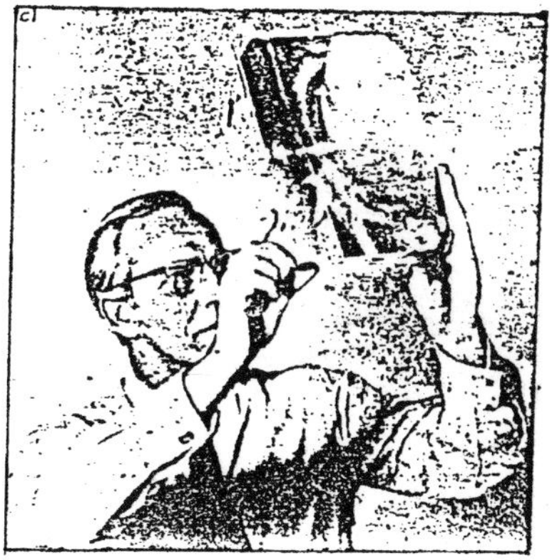

c. Pair of Freznel lenses, cemented around the edges, for overhead condenser

tungsten halogen illumination source means that it can be used in normal lecture or classroom lighting.

Focusing is effected by rotating the large focusing wheel conveniently located at the front of the instruments so that the operator does not have to stretch over the projector to focus. The friction drive movement provides a smooth positive action and can by adjusted to individual requirements.

Access to projector interior can be obtained by releasing the slide catches and lifting the top cover. This activates a safety cutout double Pole Switch which automatically cut of the electric supply.

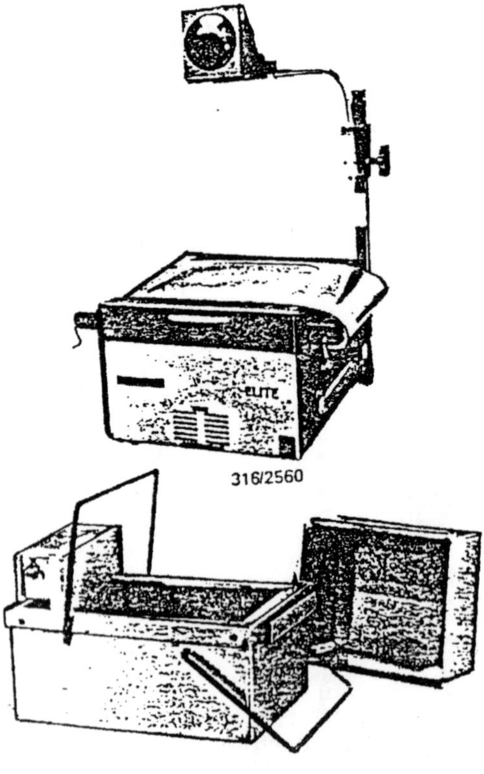

Fig. 5: Overhead Projector

The Freznel lens is easily removable for cleaning and this also permits quick cleaning for both sided of the glass screen. The tungsten halogen lamp, operating through a built-in transformer, brings all the advantages of low voltage illumination to overhead projection and eliminates the need for a heat filter.

DIRECTOR PROJECTOR:

How you wish could project write-ups, tabular datasheets, figures (and even 3-dimensional objects) directly, instead of expending time, efforts and money in getting OHP transparencies of slides? The old monstrous epidiascope was never satisfactory. However, recently direct projectors have become available for projecting documents as well as 3-D objects directly form the original into screen. One such equipment, manufactured by M/s Plus Corporation Japan, model DP-60M (Fig. 6) is described here.

The direct projector has power consumption of 950 W (220-240V AC) and has two metal halide lamps, 400 W each. The dimensions of the stage are 280x280 mm (11"x11"). The lens used has focal length f=323 mm (12.7") F2.45 and the magnification is 3 to 8 time (9 to 64 times area). The projection distance range is 1.3 to 3 meters (51"-118"). The angle of elevation is 10 to 20°. Focus is finely adjustable with main focus and auxiliary focus adjustments. Forced air cooling is provided by a fan. For safety, there is a built-in thermostat with auto reset. An auto document feeder is available optionally for convenience. The troubleshooting guide is as follow.

DATA PROJECTORS:

The data projectors which have become available in recent years offer facilities to project data, tables, figures, circuits etc. form a personal computer (PC) or laptop/notebook computer directly to screen. They it enable us to project precise images up to 300 inches across not only form the PC but also from VCR, document camera

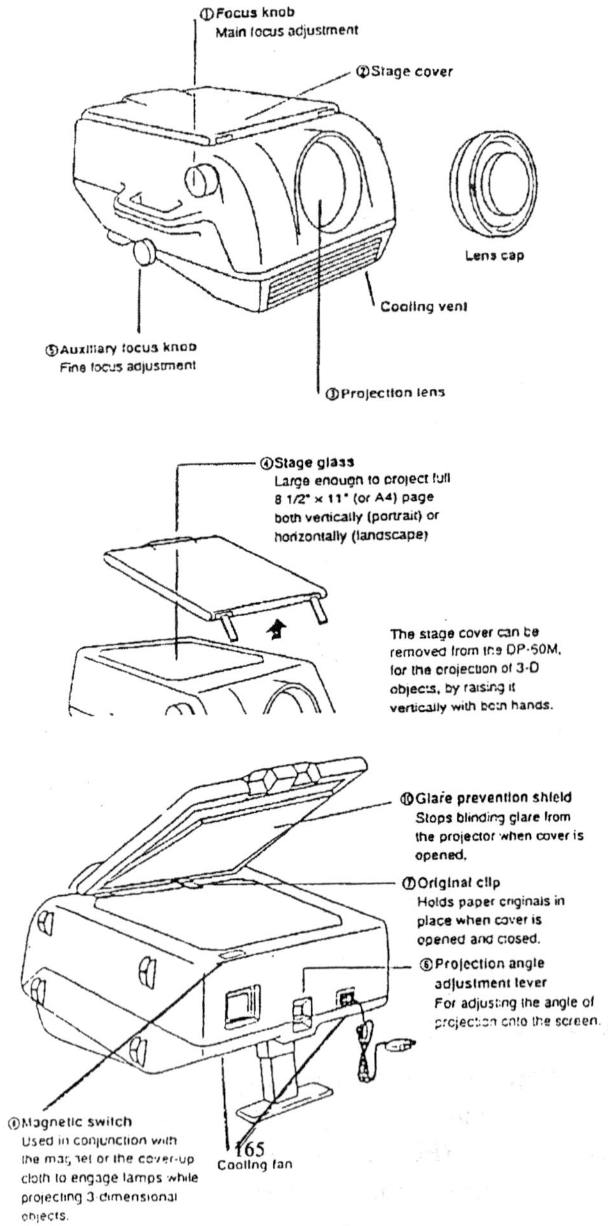

Fig. 6: DP-60M Director Projector

TROUBLESHOOTING

Before Requesting Service:

Condition	Check
Cooling fan does not run (or lamp does not light) when power switch is turned on	- Is the power plug inserted in the outlet? - Is electricity available in the outlet? - Is the lamp installed?
Lamps do not light (or only one lamp lights) when power switch is turned on	- Are the lamps not lit? Wait for 2 or 3 minutes and then turn ON the power switch. - If only one lamp is lit, wait for 1 minute before turning the unit OFF. - How long have the lamps been used? They should be replaced with new ones if the usage time exceeds 500 hours.
The projected image is blurred	- Is the focus adjusted? Adjust the focus with the main focus knob or the auxiliary focus knob. - Is the original material positioned flat on the glass? It should be brought into close contact with the stage glass.
The entire screen (or part of it) is dark lamp shutter is closed))	- Is the lens cap removed? - Are both lamps lit? - Is the stage cover help open because the object being projected is too thick? Use the blackout cloth provided.

If the units still not functioning after these checks have been made, or if you require new lamps to be installed please call plus Corporation or your local dealer.

of even a laser disc player. A remote control can be used wirelessly and we can also use the remote control with a remote mouse a receiver to operate the mouse on our PC. One such data projector, model UP-800, to manufacture by M/s Plus Corporation, Japan, is shown in Fig.7 and described here.

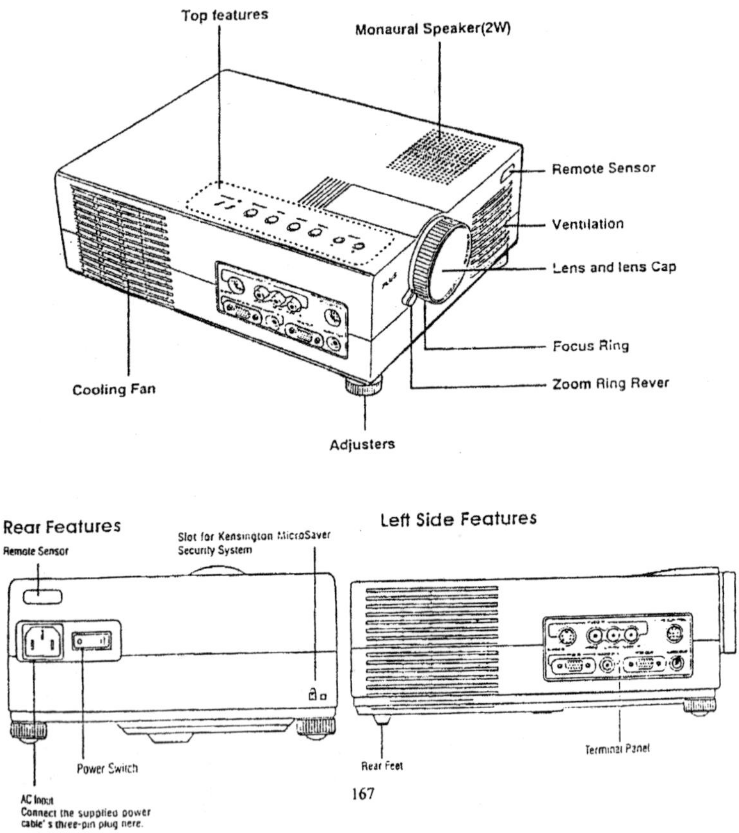

Fig. 7 UP - 800 Data Projector

UP-800 data projector incorporates a single chip digital micro device (DMD), 800X600 dots. It has manual zoom lens (with manual focus) with f=27.5-35.75 mm. The image size can be 610-7620 mm (24-300 inches). Diagonal. Projection distance range is 1.2 to 12.3 meters. The light output is 600 ANSI lumens (normally white). The lamp has a working life to 1000 hours.

The DMD and the design geometry increase the light efficiency. The 3 basic colors (RGB) can be reproduced on a single DMD, giving superior brightness, smaller size and lighter weight.

The terminal panel of UP- 800 has (i) Video input port for connecting a VCR or laser disk player or documents camera: left and right channel audio input jacks; and S-video input for connecting an external source like a VCR, (ii) RGB input connector (D-sub 15 pin) for connecting PC or other RGB equipment; and RGB audio input mini jack to connect RGB audio output form a computer. You can use your remote control wireless to operates UP-800 data projector. With the remote mouse receiver connected to you computer, you can also use the projector's remote to operate your computer's mouse wireless, too.

19

MICROTOME

Microtome are precision instruments used for cutting material into thin sections for examinations with a microscope, are also called cutting engines.

The cutting edge of an ideal microtome knife should be the straight line formed by the intersection of two planes, the cutting facets. The angle between the planes is called the bevel angle and should be greater than the wedge angle between the sides of the knife. In practice, there is a slightly radius of curvature on the edge which is approximately 0.30 μ to 0.35 μ. When the cutting edge is examined by a reflected light under 100X magnification it should appear a very fine continuous line. The proof of a sharp knife is the ability to cut a paraffin ribbon at 2 u to 3 u. The nature of the edge is also important for cutting hard or dense material.

There are two types of Microtomes:

1. With movable knife, in which the knife moves around a vertical axis.
2. With stationary knife, in which object moves along the vertical axis.

Certain functions are common to all modern microtomes and ultra microtome, although they may be performed in different ways. An arm carrying the specimen block is moved downward, a very small movement of the specimen towards the knife between each cut results a thin slice or section being detached form the face of the specimen block. Most of the microtome have two or three ranges of advance, a coarse control for initial alignment, a fine advance for cutting sections up to several microtometers thick for ultra thin sections.

The coarse control is made by moving the knife towards the specimen block, but for ultra fine advance the specimen arm is usually moved towards the knife. The cutting speed is the rate at which the specimen passes the knife during the cutting stroke and is generally expressed in millimeters per second. This speed should remain constant over a specified distance. A selection of cutting speed is required to cope with the various different consistencies and sectioning properties of different specimens.

Once a section has been cut, it normally remains attached to the knife edge, therefore the specimen block should not be allowed to pass close to the knife on its upwards return stroke or the section should be removed. Avoiding the specimen arm is deflected sideways or backwards or by refracting knife during return stroke in most of the modern microtome.

Sectioning Problems:

The following are the most common problems that may arise at the time of sectioning.

1. ***Irregular Sectioning***: If no sections are produced after the first contact, check whether the fine advance is operational check whether the fine advance is operational and has not reached the end of its travel. If sections are produced but in every stroke or the thickness of section varies with section to section, then the cutting edge is not sharp enough, which may be due to blunt knife edge.

Irregular thickness can also be caused if the knife and the specimen block are not firmly clamped in their holders or there are random movement of the specimen arm.

2. ***Poor Ribbon Formation***: if the sections do not adhere together in a ribbon, the most usual reason is that the upper and lower edges of the block face are not straight.
3. ***Sections Dragging Over Knife Edge***: This often occurs with a soft specimen block because the section is not cleanly detached from the upper edge of the block face, but it turn away leaving ragged edge.
4. ***Holes in the Section***: This is a problem of poor embedding and generally arises where there are areas of hard tissue in the specimen.
5. ***Scratches***: Any straight mark running through a series of sections perpendicular to the knife edge is due to defect in the knife edge.
6. ***Chatter***: This term chatter is used to describe the effects caused by vibrations set up in matching tools but in electron microscopy, it has come to mean the effect of a high frequency vibration set up between the knife edge and the specimen, which produces closely spaced variation in section thickness parallel to knife edge, therefore instrument should be lubricated with machine oil.
7. ***Care & Handling***: Microtome is known as cutting engine and the best result can be obtained if the specimen block or knife moves in a perfect straight line with every equispace step/strokes for which very fine uniform thread or rotating rod and the backless free up-down movement is responsible. Therefore, the instrument should be kept in a dust free room, because a single particle of dust can spoil the shared and also fine smooth movement. Instrument should be cleaned with clearing agents like kerosene or acetone and then machine oil for lubrication should be applied. Other parts like clamping screws etc. should be

checked time to time. Straight edge of knife should be saved.

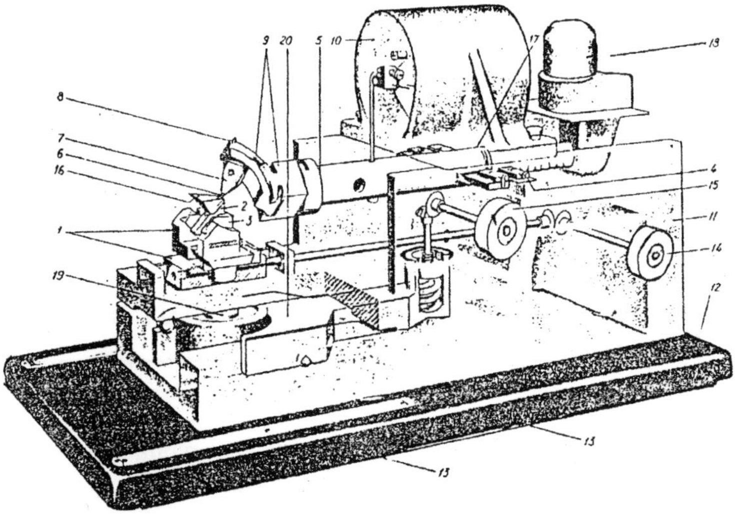

Diagrammatic representation of the LKB Ultrotomes. (1) Knife stage: (2) Glass knife: (3) Knife holder (4) Blade springs: (5) Specimen arm: (6) Specimen block: (7) Specimen holder: (8) Adjustable arch: (9) Specimen orientation head: (10) Moving - coil mechanism: (11) Foundation block: (12) Steel base-plate: (13) Damping cushions: (14) 'Macro- feed' knob: (15) 'Micro-feed' knob: (16) Collecting trough: (17) Hearing coils: (18) Blower: (19) Retraction magnet: (20) Micro-feed beam. (By courtesy of LKB Produkter AB.)

20

OVEN/ INCUBATOR, OTHER HEATING INSTRUMENTS

Experimentation under controlled condition may require controlled environment, the need of which is more keenly felt in the filed of life Sciences.

Environmental parameters such as humidity, temperature, composition of the atmosphere, etc. need to be understood and also need to be kept under tight control in the course of experimentation.

Sometimes such environment is required for the purpose of preparing sample which need to be examined under different environmental conditions.

One of the most frequently controlled environmental parameter is temperature.

The technical nature of the equipment controlling temperature will depend mostly on:-

1. Temperature at which the system/material is to be held.
2. Nature of the sample.
3. Range of temperature variations that could be permitted by the system in experiment.

Broadly the heating equipment can be categorized as follows:-

1. Ovens & Furnaces
2. Incubators
3. Constant temperature baths

OVENS & FURNACES:

Basic principle of heating equipment:–

If a current is passed through a resistor located in thermally insulated chamber, most of the heat generated is conserved and can be applied to a wide variety of heating processes.

Such insulated chambers are called Ovens of furnaces, depending on the temperature range and use.

The term oven is generally applied to units which operate upto approx. 450^0C. The term furnace generally applies to units operating above this temperature upto approx. 450°C. The term furnace gernrally applies to unit operating above the temperature upto about 1800 ^{0}C. In furnaces the thermal insulation is made up of an inner wall of fire-clay, kaolin or high-alumina or zirconia brick, depending on the temp. In addition asbestos fiber & diatomaceous earth is used as secondary insulation blocks.

Typical uses of furnaces

Heat treatment or melting of metals, glazing of ceramics, annealing glass, calcimining ores.

Typical uses of ovens

Low temperature treatment of metals, baking , drying etc.

Oven construction

For thermal insulation rock wool or glass wool is used between inner & outer steel casing.

Gravity convection models have perforated chambers floor to allow heated air to dispersion & rise quickly through the space left between the samples.

Forced convection models have forced air circulation to allow more rapid and effective heat distribution and to permit higher density work loads.

Thermometer for temperature measurement can be inserted through vent opening into the centre of chamber.

Temperature control is ON/OFF type. An energy regulartor supplies power to the heating element a certain percentage of time, depending on the setting of the control knob. No feedback relationship between the control & the temperature measured by thermometer of thermocouple. Constant supervision by the user is required at all times. Over-temperature protection should be present.

A timer can be provided to turn the oven either ON or OFF at any defined time.

LABORATORY OVEN:

Laboratory ovens are ovens for high-forced volume thermal convection applications. These ovens generally provide uniform temperatures throughout. Process applications for laboratory ovens can be for annealing, die-bond curing, drying, Polyimide baking, sterilizing, and other industrial laboratory functions. Typical sizes are from one cubic foot to 32 cubic feet (0.91 m^3) with temperatures that can be over 650 degrees fahrenheit (340 degrees celsius). Laboratory ovens can be used in numerous different applications and configurations, including clean rooms, forced convection, horizontal airflow, inert atmosphere, natural convection, and pass through. Some of the types of industries that typically use these laboratory ovens are the healthcare industry, technology industry, and transportation industry.

INCUBATOR

They are special heating systems which create environment for incubating samples in prescribed condition.

It is basically a laboratory cabinet with controlled temperature for the cultivation of bacteria or for facilitating biological tests.

Generally designed for temperatures up to 60-65 ^{0}C .

Refrigerated incubators/freezers – 100 ^{0}C to + 60 ^{0}C

Arrangements generally made to provide necessary atmosphere in the system such as O_2 or any other desired gas.

Important feature is built in temperature control to precisely control the temperature at one selected temperature. The user sets the control to the desired temperature & the chamber heats to this level, automatically. No supervision by the user is necessary.

A- Digital display may be provided to indicate the actual & set temperature at all times.

B- Non-indicating (Blind-controllers) temperature controllers do not indicate the measured temperature.

C- Programmable temperature controllers provide additional facilities such as programmed heat or cool rates, hold facility etc.

An inner glass door permits the user to open the outside door & view the contents in the chamber, while minimising heat loss.

Constant Temperature Baths : (Temperature Calibration Baths)

1. ***Constant Temperature Liquid Baths***: Immersion-type heaters.

   Liquid used: Water, Water + Ethylene Glycol, Kerosene, Silicon Oil, Hydro-Carbon, Oils etc.

Temperature range: 40°C to + 200°C

Offers highest standard in precision, reliability and versatility

2. ***Dry-block heaters***: Economical, completely dry, compact for general purpose temperature calibration.

   Temperature range: 25°C to 450°C

   Insert blocks of Al & Al-alloy with excellent thermal conductivity

   Standard rectangular/square blocks with various size holes.

3. ***Fluidized bath***: Contain a dry medium a loosely packed mass of insert particles like aluminum oxide. Through this a stream of gas is passed.

   The medium displays many of the physical properties of a liquid, but has the advantages that it cannot boil, freeze or evaporate.

   Typical temperature range: 100°C to + 1100°C

Safety:

The bath is filled with Al-oxide particles which are dry, insert, non-toxic, non corrosive, do not react violently with water, odorless. The bath is pollution-free, & no fire or explosion risks-safer to use than oil or molten metal baths.

BACTERIOLGICAL INCUBATOR:

In biology, an incubator is a device used to grow and maintain microbiological cultures or cell cultures. The incubator maintains optimal temperature, humidity and other conditions such as the carbon dioxide (CO_2) and oxygen content of the atmosphere inside. Incubators are essential for a lot of experimental work in cell biology, microbiology and molecular biology and are used to culture both bacterial as well as eukaryotic cells.

Incubators are also used in the poultry industry to act as a substitute for hens. This often results in higher hatch rates due to

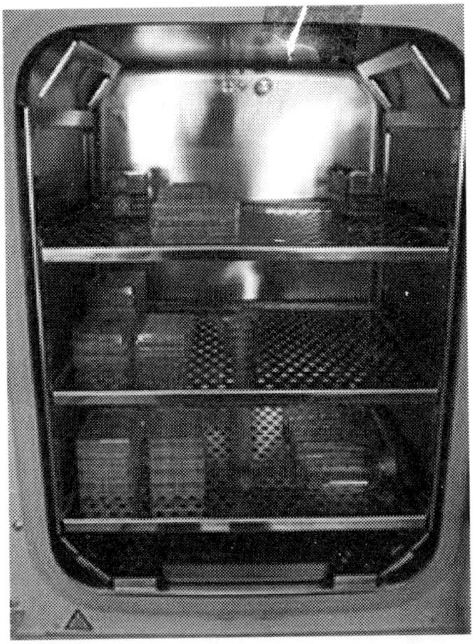

the ability to control both temperature and humidity. Various brands of incubators are commercially available to breeders.

The simplest incubators are insulated boxes with an adjustable heater, typically going up to 60 to 65°C (140 to 150°F), though some can go slightly higher (generally to no more than 100°C). The most commonly used temperature both for bacteria such as the frequently used E. Coli as well as for mammalian cells is approximately 37°C, as these organisms grow well under such conditions. For other organisms used in biological experiments, such as the budding yeast Saccharomyces cerevisiae, a growth temperature of 30°C is optimal.

More elaborate incubators can also include the ability to lower the temperature (via refrigeration), or the ability to control humidity or CO_2 levels. This is important in the cultivation of mammalian cells, where the relative humidity is typically >95% and a slightly acidic pH is achieved by maintaining a CO_2 level of 5%.

Most incubators include a timer; some can also be programmed to cycle through different temperatures, humidity levels, etc. Incubators can vary in size from tabletop to units the size of small rooms.

There are many other ways to create an incubator. The renowned scientist Louis Pasteur used the small opening underneath his staircase as an incubator.

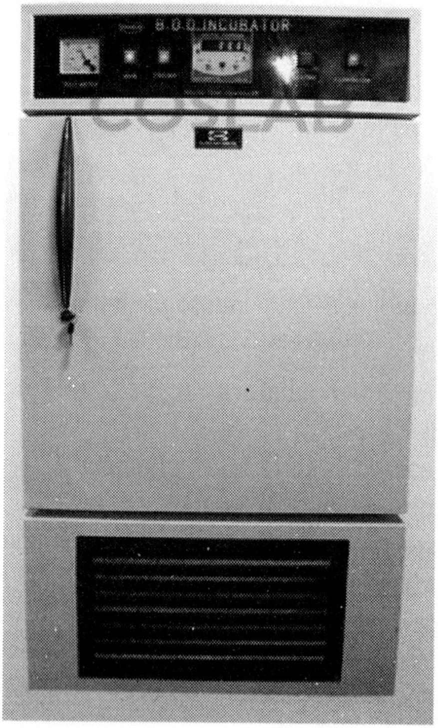

The maximum temperature for sterilization is 200°C. If a hot room is not available, it may be necessary to buy an equivalent dry incubator. Even with a hot room, it is sometimes convenient to have another incubator close to the hood for trypsinization. The incubator should be large enough, ~50–200 L (1.5–6 ft^3) per person, and should have forced-air circulation, temperature control to within ±0.2 °C, and a safety thermostat that cuts off if the incubator overheats or, better, that regulates the incubator if the first thermostat fails. The incubator should be resistant to corrosion (e.g., stainless steel, although anodized aluminum is acceptable for a dry incubator) and easily cleaned. A double chamber, or two incubators stacked, one above the other, independently regulated, is preferable to one large incubator because it can accommodate more cultures with better temperature control, and if one half fails or needs to be cleaned, the other can still be used. Many incubators have a heated water jacket to distribute heat evenly around the cabinet, thus avoiding the formation of cold spots. These incubators also hold their temperature longer in the event of a heater failure or cut in power. However, new high-efficiency insulation and diffuse surface heater elements have all but eliminated the need for a water jacket and make moving the incubator much simpler. (A water jacket generally needs to be emptied if the incubator is to be moved.) Incubator shelving is usually perforated to facilitate the circulation of air. However, the perforations can lead to irregularities in cell distribution in monolayer cultures, with variations in cell density following the pattern of spacing on the shelves. The variations may be due to convection currents generated over points of contact relative to holes in the shelf, or they may be related to areas that cool down more quickly when the door is opened. Although no problem may arise in routine maintenance, flasks and dishes should be placed on an insulated tile or metal tray in experiments in which uniform density is important.

Humid CO_2 Incubator:

Although cultures can be incubated in sealed flasks in a regular dry incubator or a hot room, some vessels, e.g., Petri dishes or multiwell plates, require a controlled atmosphere with high humidity and elevated CO_2 tension. The cheapest way of controlling the gas phase is to place the cultures in a plastic box, or chamber (Bellco, MP Biomedicals): Gas the container with the correct CO_2 mixture and then seal it. If the container is not completely filled with dishes, include an open dish of water to increase the humidity inside the chamber. CO_2 incubators are more expensive, but their case of use and superior control of CO_2 tension and temperature (anaerobic jars and desiccators take longer to warm up) justify the expenditure. A controlled atmosphere is achieved by using a humidifying tray and controlling the CO_2 tension with a CO_2-monitoring device, which draws air from the incubator into a sample chamber, determines the concentration of CO_2, and injects pure CO_2 into the incubator to make up any deficiency. Air is circulated around the incubator by natural convection or by using a fan to keep both the CO_2 level and the temperature uniform. It is claimed that fan-circulated incubators recover faster after opening, although natural convection incubators can still have a quick recovery and greatly reduce the risks of contamination. Dry, heated wall incubators also encourage less fungal contamination on the walls, as the walls tend to remain dry, even at high relative humidity. Some CO_2 controllers need to be calibrated every few months, but the use of gold wire or infrared detectors minimizes drift and many models reset the zero of the CO_2 detector automatically. The size of incubator required will depend on usage, both the numbers of people using it and the types of cultures. Five people using only microtitration plates could have 1000 plates (100,000 individual cultures) or 10 experiments each in a modest-size dincubator, while one person doing cell cloning could fill one shelf with one or two experiments. Flask cultures, especially large flasks, are not an economical use of CO_2 incubators. They are better incubated in a regular incubator or hot room. If CO_2 is required, flasks can be gassed from a cylinder or CO_2 supply.

LAMINAR AIR FLOW:

A laminar flow cabinet or laminar air flow closet or tissue culture hood is a carefully enclosed bench designed to prevent contamination of semiconductor wafers, biological samples, or any particle sensitive device. Air is drawn through a HEPA filter and blown in a very smooth, laminar air flow towards the user. The cabinet is usually made of stainless steel with no gaps or joints where spores might collect.

Such hoods exist in both horizontal and vertical configurations, and there are many different types of cabinets with a variety of airflow patterns and acceptable uses. NSF49 is the commonly accepted regulatory standard for these cabinets.

Laminar Air flow cabinets may have a UV-C germicidal lamp to sterilize the shell and contents when not in use. (It is important to switch this light off during use, as it will quickly give any exposed skin sunburn and may cause cataracts.

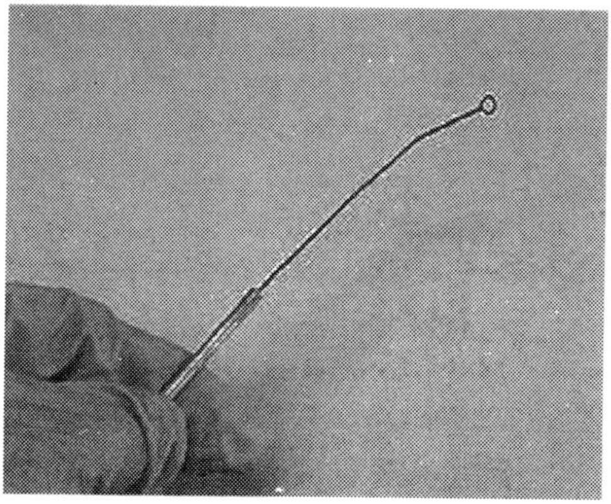

INOCULATION LOOP:

An inoculation loop, also called a smear loop, inoculation wand or microstreaker, is a simple tool used mainly by microbiologists to retrieve an inoculum from a culture of microorganisms. The loop is used in the cultivation of microbes on plates by transferring inoculum for streaking.

The wire forms a small loop with a diameter of about 5 mm. The loop of wire at the tip may be made of platinum or nichrome, the latter being inferior but less expensive. This loop removes a consistent amount of the liquid suspended inoculum by using the phenomenon of surface tension.

The inoculation loop is sterilized in a flame until it becomes red hot before and after each use. By doing this, the same tool can be reused in different experiments without fear of cross-contamination. After flame sterilization, the loop must be cooled so that the next cells the loop touches are not killed by the hot metal.

***

INDEX

L

M

N

O

P

Q

R

S

T

U